Obesity in Orthopedics

Guest Editor

GEORGE V. RUSSELL, MD

ORTHOPEDIC CLINICS OF NORTH AMERICA

www.orthopedic.theclinics.com

January 2011 • Volume 42 • Number 1

SAUNDERS an imprint of ELSEVIER, Inc.

W.B. SAUNDERS COMPANY
A Division of Elsevier Inc.

1600 John F. Kennedy Blvd. • Suite 1800 • Philadelphia, PA 19103-2899.

http://www.orthopedic.theclinics.com

ORTHOPEDIC CLINICS OF NORTH AMERICA Volume 42, Number 1
January 2011 ISSN 0030-5898, ISBN-13: 978-1-4557-0478-1

Editor: Debora Dellapena

Orthopedic Clinics of North America (ISSN 0030-5898) is published quarterly by Elsevier Inc., 360 Park Avenue South, New York, NY 10010-1710. Months of issue are January, April, July, and October. Business and Editorial Offices: 1600 John F. Kennedy Blvd., Suite 1800, Philadelphia, PA 19103-2899. Customer Service Office: 3251 Riverport Lane, Maryland Heights, MO 63043. Periodicals postage paid at New York, NY and additional mailing offices. Subscription prices are $269.00 per year for (US individuals), $513.00 per year for (US institutions), $318.00 per year (Canadian individuals), $615.00 per year (Canadian institutions), $392.00 per year (international individuals), $615.00 per year (international institutions), $132.00 per year (US students), $191.00 per year (Canadian and international students). Foreign air speed delivery is included in all *Clinics* subscription prices. All prices are subject to change without notice. **POSTMASTER:** Send change of address to *Orthopedic Clinics of North America*, **Elsevier Health Sciences Division, Subscription Customer Service, 3251 Riverport Lane, Maryland Heights, MO 63043. Customer Service (orders, claims, online, change of address): Elsevier Health Sciences Division, Subscription Customer Service, 3251 Riverport Lane, Maryland Heights, MO 63043. Tel: 1-800-654-2452 (U.S. and Canada); 314-447-8871 (outside U.S. and Canada). Fax: 314-447-8029. E-mail: journalscustomerservice-usa@elsevier. com (for print support); journalsonlinesupport-usa@elsevier.com (for online support).**

Reprints. For copies of 100 or more, of articles in this publication, please contact the Commercial Reprints Department, Elsevier Inc., 360 Park Avenue South, New York, NY 10010-1710. Tel.: 212-633-3812; Fax: 212-462-1935; E-mail: reprints@elsevier. com.

Orthopedic Clinics of North America is covered in *MEDLINE/PubMed* (*Index Medicus*), *Cinahl, Excerpta Medica,* and *Cumulative Index to Nursing and Allied Health Literature.*

Printed and bound by CPI Group (UK) Ltd, Croydon, CR0 4YY

Transferred to Digital Print 2011

Contributors

GUEST EDITOR

GEORGE V. RUSSELL, MD
Associate Professor, Department of
Orthopaedic Surgery, University of Mississippi
Medical Center, Jackson, Mississippi

AUTHORS

DANIEL T. ALTMAN, MD
Associate Professor of Orthopaedic Surgery,
Department of Orthopaedic Surgery, Allegheny
General Hospital, Pittsburgh; Drexel University
College of Medicine, Philadelphia,
Pennsylvania

PETER BATES, FRCS(Orth)
Barts and the London NHS Trust, Whitechapel,
London, United Kingdom

VICTORIA A. CATENACCI, MD
Assistant Professor of Medicine, Division of
Endocrinology, Diabetes, and Metabolism,
Department of Medicine, University of
Colorado Denver, Denver, Colorado

SONIA CHAUDHRY, MD
Resident-Physician, Department of
Orthopaedic Surgery, New York University
Hospital for Joint Diseases, New York,
New York

KENNETH A. EGOL, MD
Professor and Vice-Chairman, Department of
Orthopaedic Surgery, New York University
Hospital for Joint Diseases, New York,
New York

STEVEN L. FRICK, MD
Residency Director, Department of
Orthopaedic Surgery, Carolinas Medical
Center, Charlotte, North Carolina

MICHAEL J. GARDNER, MD
Assistant Professor, Orthopaedic Trauma
Service, Department of Orthopaedic Surgery,
Washington University School of Medicine,
St. Louis, Missouri

JOSHUA GARY, MD
Department of Orthopaedic Surgery, University
of Texas Southwestern Medical Center,
Dallas, Texas

F. KEITH GETTYS, MD
Resident, Department of Orthopaedic Surgery,
Carolinas Medical Center, Charlotte,
North Carolina

MATT L. GRAVES, MD
Associate Director, Residency Program;
Assistant Professor, Division of Trauma,
Department of Orthopaedic Surgery and
Rehabilitation, University of Mississippi
Medical Center, Jackson, Mississippi

ROBERT M. GREENLEAF, MD
Resident Orthopaedic Surgery, Allegheny
General Hospital, Pittsburgh, Pennsylvania

BRIAN R. HAMLIN, MD
Associate Director, The Orthopedic Program,
Magee Womens Hospital of University of
Pittsburgh Medical Center, Pittsburgh, PA

J. BENJAMIN JACKSON, MD
Resident, Department of Orthopaedic Surgery,
Carolinas Medical Center, Charlotte,
North Carolina

CLIFFORD B. JONES, MD, FACS
Department of Surgery, College of Human
Medicine, Michigan State University;
Adjunct Professor, Van Andel Institute;
Orthopaedic Associates of Michigan,
Grand Rapids, Michigan

MADHAV A. KARUNAKAR, MD
Orthopaedic Traumatologist, Department of Orthopaedic Surgery, Carolinas Medical Center, Charlotte, North Carolina

ROBERT K. MEHRLE, MD
Assistant Professor, Department of Orthopedic Surgery and Rehabilitation, University of Mississippi Medical Center, Jackson, Mississippi

LOREN NUNLEY, BA
Medical Student, Howard University College of Medicine, Washington, District of Columbia

CHRISTINE W. PIERCE, MD
Resident, Department of Orthopaedic Surgery, University of Mississippi Medical Center, Jackson, Mississippi

SCOTT E. PORTER, MD
Section Chief, Division of Orthopaedic Oncology, Department of Orthopaedic Surgery, Greenville Hospital System, University Medical Center, Greenville, South Carolina

CHARLES REINERT, MD
Department of Orthopaedic Surgery, University of Texas Southwestern Medical Center, Dallas, Texas

WILLIAM M. RICCI, MD
Professor and Chief, Orthopaedic Trauma Service, Department of Orthopaedic Surgery, Washington University School of Medicine, St. Louis, Missouri

GEORGE V. RUSSELL, MD
Associate Professor, Department of Orthopaedic Surgery, University of Mississippi Medical Center, Jackson, Mississippi

GURPREET SINGH, MD
Department of Orthopaedic Surgery, University of Texas Southwestern Medical Center, Dallas, Texas

ADAM STARR, MD
Department of Orthopaedic Surgery, University of Texas Southwestern Medical Center, Dallas, Texas

PHILIPP N. STREUBEL, MD
Clinical Research Fellow, Orthopaedic Trauma Service, Department of Orthopaedic Surgery, Washington University School of Medicine, St. Louis, Missouri

SCOTT A. WINGERTER, MD, PhD
Resident Physician, Department of Orthopedic Surgery and Rehabilitation, University of Mississippi Medical Center, Jackson, Mississippi

Contents

injuries in the obese population, the suggestions that are provided are based on the extrapolation from published evidence of fracture care in other areas in patients with obesity, logic, and personal experience with fracture care in patients with obesity.

Ankle fractures are a common orthopedic injury. Certain ankle injuries have been associated with patient demographics such as obesity and smoking. Obese patients are more prone to severe ankle injuries. Naturally, these injuries affect the lower extremity mobility significantly, which itself is a risk factor for obesity. Although obese patients have increased complications across the board, there are specific techniques that can be used to assure the best possible outcome. The perioperative, surgical, and postoperative considerations as well as the outcomes are discussed in this article.

A body mass index (BMI) greater than 30 is becoming increasingly common in the United States. Surgery for pelvic and acetabular fractures in this population is particularly problematic because conventional treatment often requires large surgical exposures. The surgery for both these fractures is technically difficult because of the volume of soft tissue and proneness to complications. Wound problems and infections are particularly common after open surgery in obese patients, and these increase linearly with the BMI. In this article, we present a small consecutive series over 14 months on obese patients who underwent percutaneous treatment of their pelvic or acetabular fractures.

The open operative management of pelvic and acetabular fractures in the obese is technically demanding, with a significantly higher rate of complications compared with patients who are nonobese. The decision to perform surgery should involve a thorough understanding of risks, and patients should be counseled. Careful attention should be paid to patient factors; coexisting systemic conditions and patient positioning to reduce complications. Wound complications are most commonly seen, and techniques to reduce risk should be incorporated. When complications occur, aggressive management can result in successful salvage. Future areas of study should include methods to reduce risk of surgical site infections and improving our understanding of the physiologic alterations that occur with obesity. This article summarizes the current literature on open treatment of pelvic and acetabular fractures in the obese patient, reviews the physiologic adaptations of obesity as they relate to pelvic surgery, highlights risk factors for complications, and provides recommendations to reduce the incidence of complications.

Given the increasing incidence and severity of obesity in the adult population, orthopaedic surgeons are evaluating and treating more acutely injured obese patients. Management of obese patients is complicated given their body habitus and associated medical comorbidities. Although evaluation and treatment are almost the same as for nonobese patients, some special considerations are necessary to prevent errors in diagnosis and treatment of obese trauma patients. This article focuses on spine injuries in obese patients. Predisposition to spinal injury, effective evaluation and early management, principles of treatment planning, operative technical pearls, and postoperative management are discussed.

Obesity is a rapidly expanding health problem in children and adolescents and is the most prevalent nutritional problem for children in the United States. Some believe that obesity has become a major epidemic in American children, with the prevalence having more than doubled since 1980. This epidemic has led to a near-doubling in hospitalizations with a diagnosis of obesity between 1999 and 2005 and an increase in costs from $125.9 million to $237.6 million between 2001 and 2005. This article describes some of the orthopaedic conditions commonly encountered in overweight/obese children and adolescents, classically infantile and adolescent tibia vara and slipped capital femoral epiphysis. Also discussed are genu valgum, which has been associated with obesity, and other difficulties encountered in providing orthopaedic care to obese children.

The purpose of this article is to present the challenges of dealing with the morbidly obese patient suffering from degenerative knee arthrosis. Surgery should only be undertaken when conservative management has failed and comorbidities optimized. Owing to risks related to comorbidities, diligence is necessary before proceeding with surgery to lessen the chance of complications—especially infection. Evaluation, conservative treatments, preoperative optimization, and surgical options are discussed.

There has been a significant increase in the prevalence of obesity in the United States over the last 20 years, with the highest percentage in Mississippi. The percentage of obese patients undergoing total hip arthroplasty (THA) appears to be increasing at an even faster rate. Orthopedic surgeons performing hip arthroplasty need to be aware of potential issues to minimize complications associated with this population. This article outlines preoperative and postoperative care and describes current techniques and tools used by surgeons in obese patients to facilitate soft tissue dissection, exposure, implant placement, and closure.

The obesity epidemic continues to grow. As the number of obese people increases, it is logical to expect an increasing number of obese patients and increasing costs to care for these patients. Orthopedic surgeons will see many of these patients who need treatment for injuries and chronic conditions. Care of obese patients requires more work and time in providing nonoperative and operative care. No system has been proposed to handle reimbursement disparities, particularly for providers. The model for health care will change and, along with it, should be all parties coming together to address inequalities and inequities in care for obese and morbidly obese patients.

Orthopedic Clinics of North America

THE CLINICS ARE NOW AVAILABLE ONLINE!

Access your subscription at:
www.theclinics.com

Preface
Obesity in Orthopedics

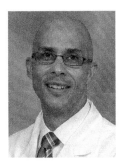

George V. Russell, MD
Guest Editor

The obesity epidemic is ever increasing, not only in the United States, but throughout the rest of the world. As the population increases in size, it is only reasonable to assume that our patients will be larger. This edition of *Orthopedic Clinics of North America* is specifically dedicated to the challenges of treating obese and morbidly obese patients.

The authors live and work primarily in those states with the highest concentration of obesity. Due to their practice locations, the authors have particular expertise in managing obese patients within their particular specialty areas. Other authors, not in the most obese states, have an interest in obese patients and have previously written scholarly work about the effects of obesity.

Not all specialties are affected equally by obesity; therefore, we included those areas that have been negatively associated with obesity. The aim of this issue is to highlight those practice areas most impacted by obesity such as arthroplasty of the lower extremity, pediatric concerns, and the impact of caring for patients with both common and uncommon fractures. There is even an article that educates the reader about office space and equipment concerns with a very moving section addressing biases toward obese patients.

Working in the most obese state in the nation, Mississippi, I have developed a keen appreciation for the challenges and difficulties of treating obese and morbidly obese patients. I expect my coauthors and I will make you aware of the overall obesity epidemic and its impact upon orthopedics. We will all be impacted by obesity in our practices. My challenge to the readers is to embrace the following articles and use them to guide compassionate care for this segment of our patient population.

I am indebted to all of my coauthors for their time and expertise. A special thanks is also due to the many residents who have worked side by side with me through the years on our patients. I also wish to thank Debora Dellapena, who made all this possible.

George V. Russell, MD
Department of Orthopaedic Surgery
University of Mississippi Medical Center
2500 North State Street
Jackson, MS 39216, USA

E-mail address:
gvrussell@umc.edu

Orthop Clin N Am 42 (2011) ix
doi:10.1016/j.ocl.2010.09.004

Office and Hospital Needs

Scott E. Porter, MD[a],*, Victoria A. Catenacci, MD[b]

KEYWORDS
- Obesity • Morbid obesity • Magnetic resonance
- Computed tomography • Orthopedic surgery

Obesity as a medical condition is currently at historic epidemiologic levels and is rising.[1] It has been proven to affect nearly every facet of medical care from the delivery of this care to its reception. Patients who are obese present novel challenges to each and every surgeon. Historically, these patients and their body habitués were anomalies whose orthopedic care admittedly differed from that of their lean counterparts for a variety of reasons. With the current national trends in obesity, however, this segment of the population has increased dramatically. Overweight and obese patients will increasingly seek routine, traumatic, urgent, and emergent orthopedic care and every orthopedic surgeon should be adequately prepared to treat overweight and obese patients.

EPIDEMIOLOGY

Obesity has come to be clinically and epidemiologically defined by one's body mass index (BMI).[2] A person's BMI is calculated by dividing his or her weight as measured in kilograms (kg) by the square of his or her height, measured in meters (m^2). **Table 1** shows the categories of BMI. A healthy BMI range is 18.5 to 24.9 kg/m^2. Overweight is defined as a BMI from 25.0 to 29.9 kg/m^2 and obesity is defined as BMI of 30 kg/m^2 or greater.[3] Obesity can further be subdivided based on subclasses of BMI, as shown in **Table 1**. Extreme obesity is defined as a BMI greater than 40 kg/m^2. The World Health Organization (WHO)

recently stated that obesity has reached epidemic proportions all over the world.[4] WHO estimates that more than 1 billion adults worldwide are overweight and 300 million of those people are obese. Obesity levels vary widely among nations with a prevalence of less than 5% in China, Japan, and certain African nations and a prevalence of greater than 75% in urban Samoa.[4] Even in countries with a low overall obesity rate, this rate can approach 20% in their more urban cities. Seemingly, as the income, technology, and quality of lives of a particular group of people increase, so does the obesity rate.

In the United States, there has been a dramatic rise in obesity rates since the 1980s.[2,5,6] Between 1980 and 2004 the prevalence of obesity more than doubled in American adults.[2] The most recent national estimates from the National Health and Nutrition Examination Survey (NHANES) 2007–2008 suggest that 68% of the American population is overweight and nearly 34% are obese.[7] The greatest relative increase over time has been in the proportion of severely obese individuals. The percentage of the population with a BMI of 40 or greater has increased from 0.9% in the 1960s to its current percentage of about 6%.[7] Mexican American and non-Hispanic black women currently have the highest rates of obesity (BMI ≥30) at 45% and nearly 50%, respectively. The prevalence of obesity is greater than 30% in all ethnic groups, however, and in almost all age and gender subgroups of US adults.

The authors have nothing to disclose.
No funding sources were used.
[a] Division of Orthopaedic Oncology, Department of Orthopaedic Surgery, Greenville Hospital System, University Medical Center, 2nd floor Support Tower, 701 Grove Road, Greenville, SC 29605, USA
[b] Division of Endocrinology, Diabetes, and Metabolism, Department of Medicine, University of Colorado Denver, 4455 East 12th Avenue, Denver, CO 80220, USA
* Corresponding author.
E-mail address: sporter@ghs.org

Orthop Clin N Am 42 (2011) 1–9
doi:10.1016/j.ocl.2010.07.005

Table 1
Categories of body mass index (BMI)

	Class	BMI (kg/m^2)
Underweight		<18.5
Normal weight		18.5–24.9
Overweight		25.0–29.9
Obese	I	30.0–34.9
	II	35.0–39.9
Extreme Obesity	III	≥40.0

As of 2008, the Centers for Disease Control and Prevention (CDC) estimates that only 1 of the 50 states (Colorado) has an obesity rate under 20%.[8] Although Mississippi is the perennial leader in obese statistics with nearly 33% of its population being obese, there are 5 additional states with an incidence of obesity equal to or greater than 30%. Flegal and colleagues[7] recently interpreted results of the NHANES 1999–2008 that examine national obesity trends. The investigators have concluded that the increases in the prevalence of obesity previously observed do not appear to be continuing at the same rate as in past years. Obesity rates have increased by only about 5% in men and have remained largely statistically stagnant in women over the past decade.[7] They determined that the obesity rate among all adult women was 35.5% and the rate among men was 32.2% in 2008. Thus, depending on the practice location and focus, today's orthopedic surgeon can expect that at least one third or more of their patient population will be obese and there is no indication that rates of obesity are decreasing.

WEIGHT BIAS IN THE HEALTH CARE SETTING

Although the past several decades have seen tremendous gains in the previously pervasive stigmas surrounding race, religion, and sexuality, these advances have not yet reached weight bias.[9–13] Recent evidence suggests weight discrimination is highly prevalent in American society and has increased by 66% over the past decade.[14] The prevalence of weight discrimination is now thought to be comparable with that of race discrimination.[12] As an example, Latner and colleagues[9] comparatively researched biases held by nearly 400 university students toward "Muslim," "fat," or "gay" individuals. In reviewing their data, the investigators were able to conclude that weight bias is significantly more pervasive than the other biases within the study population. Despite the shame and prejudice induced by the weight stigma, there is a perception that weight stigmatization is justifiable and may motivate individuals to adopt healthier behaviors.[15] Rather, Puhl and Heuer[16] have concluded that stigmatization of obese individuals poses serious risks to their psychological and physical health, generates health disparities, and interferes with implementation of effective obesity prevention efforts.

Research is accumulating that obese individuals experience weight stigma in the health care setting, and that this bias may undermine obese patients' opportunity to receive effective medical care.[10,15,16] In a recent review of the English literature with its focus being the perceived attitude of nurses toward obese patients, the investigators concluded that some nurses held a perception of physical and social unattractiveness of obese patients.[17] The obese patients were at times seen to be emotionally and physically demanding. A number of negative stereotypes were held about the obese individuals, including a belief that they were disproportionately lazy and self-indulgent. Studies have also suggested that the weight of patients significantly affects how medical providers might treat them. Providers may spend less time with obese patients and may provide less health education to these patients as compared with thinner patients.[18,19] More than half of the 620 primary care doctors questioned in a study by Puhl and Brownell[20] described obese patients as "awkward, unattractive, ugly, and unlikely to comply with treatment." It is therefore not surprising that obese individuals frequently report experiences of weight bias in health care.[10,21,22]

The data presented suggest that a critical need in the treatment of the obese orthopedic patient lies in the realm of sensitivity and understanding. Orthopedic surgeons are ill-equipped to address the multifactorial nature of these challenges.[23] Kristeller and Hoerr[23] evaluated physician biases toward obese patients comparatively across 6 subspecialty fields. The results of their survey suggested that orthopedic surgeons were generally regarded as less interested in taking on any responsibility for patient weight loss management and were the least likely to provide any active intervention. Despite this, a number of orthopedic surgeons in elective practices have informal policies that encourage preoperative weight loss in potential operative candidates. A thorough search of the literature failed to find any scientific basis for this policy. There are a number of studies in the bariatric surgery literature that point to a clear benefit from preoperative weight loss in perioperative surgical parameters (ie, blood loss and surgical time), ease of surgery, and postoperative weight loss.[24–26] Results of studies like these, however, should be cautiously extrapolated to nonbariatric weight-loss surgery. Moreover, in light of the overwhelming literature that presents obese patients as a segment of society that feels continuously ostracized, an approach such as this may further degrade the health care provider–to-patient relationship. Efforts may be better served to provide an environment that allows the obese patient to feel welcomed and integrated into the mainstream patient population.

Our population of patients continues to age and to grow in any of a number of weight metrics. Kaminsky and Gadaleta[27] suggest that the medical community as a whole is seemingly prepared for the elderly, but not for the obese. They note that the absence of having the simplest and most basic of medical equipment in a size that can accommodate a larger patient can be seen as a significant lack of consideration. One must bear in mind that this occurs in a segment of the population that already harbors feelings of inadequacy, dependence, depression, and overt personality disorders at a rate that exceeds the general population.[10,27–29] Obese patients may therefore feel discriminated against, whether intentionally or not, by failures to prepare for their care or failures to recognize their needs during episodes of health care delivery.[30]

To this end, there are some key items that may help to provide an environment for obese patients that may lessen their apprehension and lack of emotional and psychological comfort.[27] An example of a simple intervention that may help to approach a reluctant obese patient and may show some forethought is having a small inventory of examination gowns that will accommodate larger patients that is kept in an area that is readily and discretely accessible.

OFFICE SPECIAL NEEDS

Obesity-related durable goods might result in significant capital expense. They may, however, prove to be invaluable during the assessment of obese patients and essential to providing for the needs of these individuals. Blood pressure assessment is nearly ubiquitous as a component of new patient examinations in the orthopedic outpatient setting. For patients who are obviously above or below the "average" weight, the standard cuff likely already attached to the sphygmomanometer may not be appropriate. The rise in obesity among our population has resulted in a necessary rise in the arm circumferences of the routine patient. Graves and colleagues[31] evaluated the NHANES data looking specifically at changes in the arm circumferences of the participants. They concluded that the average arm circumference is statistically increasing in size and that this difference is likely attributable to our increasing obesity rates. The investigators predicted that nearly 1 in 4 adults were no longer able to have their blood pressure taken with a standard adult cuff. The official guidelines for blood pressure cuff sizing suggests that a standard adult cuff (ie, 16 × 30 cm) can be used for arm circumferences 27 to 34 cm. For arm circumferences 35 to 44 cm, a large adult cuff (16 × 36 cm) should be used and for arm circumferences 45 to 52 cm, an adult thigh cuff (16 × 42 cm) should be used.[32,33] It stands to reason that having alternatively sized blood pressure cuffs readily available and seemingly in routine use may promote an environment that suggests a simple acceptance of the obvious physical differences that the obese body habitus presents.

One of the most critical durable goods in the orthopedic outpatient setting is the wheelchair. Patient ambulation is often impaired by injury, ailment, or iatrogenic causes. As the population has grown more obese, so too have their central or truncal dimensions.[34–36] Between 1988 and 1994 and 2003 and 2004, Li and colleagues[34] calculated that the mean American waist circumference had increased from 96.0 cm to 100.4 cm among men ($P<.001$) and from 89.0 cm to 94.0 cm among women ($P<.001$). The investigators furthermore deduced that more than one-half of US adults had abdominal obesity in the period of 2003 to 2004 with the criteria for abdominal obesity having been established as waist circumferences greater than 102 cm and 88 cm respectively for men and women.[34] These changes necessarily require a larger wheelchair to accommodate the girth of our larger Americans with waist circumferences above the mean. Although the International Standards Organization (ISO) governs wheelchair manufacturing, the details of sizing are quite variable.[37] The wheelchair industry has arrived at a standard seating width of 18 in. This is very similar to the 17-in standard seat width of most major American airlines.[38] To allow adequate room on either side of the seated patient for comfort, 14-in may represent a maximum patient diameter or width for standard chairs. This would clearly alienate a not so insignificant number of possible patients and inconvenience even more. In contrast, bariatric equipment manufacturers make wheelchairs in widths that surpass a 32-in seating area. Having readily available wheelchairs with expanded seating widths will again aid in providing an environment in which an obese patient may feel welcome. One must exercise some caution, however, because existing interior doorways may allow passage of only 30-in and exterior doorways may maximally allow a 36-in width. For new construction or renovations, the Americans with Disability Act Accessibility Guidelines state that the minimum required width for hallways to safely allow passage of a standard wheelchair must be 36-in continuously with 32-in allowed at any one point (ie, door jamb).[39] Again, however, these measurements are based on a standard-sized wheelchair with a standard seating width of 18-in. The increasing space needs of obese patients and the wheelchair sizes that they require necessitate wider hallways and doorjambs.

Although professional office furniture standards and codes will undoubtedly differ between cities and regions, there are some general themes that one can incorporate that may help to promote a more receptive and safer office environment for the obese patient. Seating surfaces have generally been constructed with the average lean American as the target consumer. In an ambulatory office setting, chairs without arms and loveseats can comfortably accommodate a wide range of body habitus without stigmatizing the occupant.[40]

Once a patient is in the examination room, health care providers should have some confidence that the examination table will support the heaviest of patients. Examination table manufacturer Web sites may have useful information about the weight limits of their products. Additionally, examination tables that have overhangs or "lips" may need to be bolted to the floor to prevent them from tipping over with the eccentric load imposed by obese patients with their initial attempts to sit on it.[40] A useful recommendation for providers that have input into the design of new or renovated outpatient care areas may be to designate a single room for the evaluation of the challenging patient.[40] This challenge may not be imposed by just the weight of the patient but also by patients confined to a stretcher, some elderly patients, combative patients, or difficult patients who require significant assistance otherwise. This room can be equipped with an extra-wide examination table that has been properly secured, larger gowns, and larger blood pressure cuffs and the doorway can be made with an opening of at least 36 in to accommodate stretchers and extra-wide wheelchairs alike. Additionally, this same forethought can be exercised in designing or redesigning one of the facility's

restrooms to have reinforced safety bars and an elevated commode that can be used by obese patients, elderly patients, and patients with limited mobility.

When taken as a whole, recommendations to assist in the outpatient care of obese patients have as their goals promoting an environment in which obese patients feel comfortable presenting and contributing to their care and an environment that promotes the safe and complete evaluation of the patient in question (**Table 2**). This can be obtained with foresight, an understanding of the limits of currently owned medical devices and paraphernalia, and a willingness to entertain products that will accommodate the larger American body habitus when the need for new equipment and durable goods arises.

HOSPITAL SPECIAL NEEDS

Whether the admission of obese or morbidly obese patients is scheduled or emergent, their needs should be taken into account no less than

Table 2
Listing of potentially useful outpatient facility needs

Sensitivity	Working knowledge of location of items routinely used in bariatric assessment • Thigh or oversized blood pressure cuff • Oversized hospital gowns Current listing of institutions that can accommodate bariatric imaging needs
Office needs	Furniture with wider seating surfaces or seating surfaces without arms Wheelchair with wider seating surfaces Tables that are without overhangs or are bolted to the floor Door jambs and hallways that will allow passage of wider, bariatric wheelchairs
Pearl	Designate a single room in the outpatient setting as the room for patients with special needs. This may include bariatric patients, polytrauma patients, those patients confined to a stretcher, or those patients who require more assistance than is routinely needed.

in the outpatient setting. Many of the same suggestions rendered for the ambulatory environment can be extrapolated to the inpatient environment. This includes oversized or thigh blood pressure cuffs, larger hospital gowns, furniture within the hospital rooms for visitors and guests that will accommodate the larger stature of morbidly obese family members and friends, and hallway and door jamb widths that will accommodate oversized wheelchairs, stretchers, and hospital beds. There are additional inpatient items that may aid in the safe care of obese patients (**Table 3**). These include oversized walkers and commodes; hospital beds with a variety of mattress options; and equipment to aid in the positioning, rolling, lifting, and transferring of the preoperative or postoperative morbidly obese patient.[41] With the increase in the numbers of surgeries being performed that are dedicated to the treatment of morbid obesity and/or its complications, the number of major vendors that supply bariatric lines of equipment and the variety of equipment available continue to increase.[41–44] For example, bariatric beds are usually included within the larger market for specialty beds that include beds for patients needing pulmonary care, wound care, and vascular care.[41] These beds are usually not only equipped to allow heavier weight limits and wider laying surfaces, but they usually have specialized air mattresses that aid in distributing and lessening high pressure areas that may develop in obese patients with restricted mobility.[41,45] Patients who are not extremely obese may be sufficiently serviced with a specialty bed designed with another purpose in mind.[41] It should be noted, however, that there are some data to suggest that obesity is protective against the development of pressure ulcers.[45,46] These interventions may, therefore, be more beneficial in providing a safer and more-comfortable environment than reducing a true pressure ulcer formation risk. In lieu of expensive equipment that may aid in the overall care of the obese or morbidly obese patient, it may be prudent to ensure that adequate staff is available to assist with performing these patient care activities.

Motorized tables are also quite common in the radiology department as part of magnetic resonance imaging (MRI) or computed tomography (CT) scanners. These tables may accommodate the physical size of a patient, but not their weight owing to the limitations imposed by the motor responsible for table movement. The newest generation of CT scans have bore sizes that exceed 80 cm and have beds with weight limits above 600 lb.[47,48] Although these scans may not be in routine use in the outpatient center, they may be available at regional or local medical centers. Having the location of these larger scanners as part of the outpatient staff's working knowledge may lessen the potential stigmatizing chaos that ensues when it is realized that a patient will not be accommodated by a facility's current equipment. Magnetic resonance imagers have a bore size that is critical to the image quality and therefore generally are not as spacious as CT scan bores. The bore size of most MRI machines is 60 cm (ie, 23.6 in) and the weight limit may not exceed 350 lb in even the newest generation of units. It is therefore likely that there are a number of patients whose total body diameters including their arms at their sides approaches or exceeds this measurement regardless of their weight. As the available potential space surrounding a patient decreases, noncompliance with completion of the study may increase. So too, the image quality may suffer greatly. Claustrophobia is a fear of confinement that is related to fears of suffocation and restriction.[49] In the obese patient, the fear of restriction may be a reality. Although there has been no study to date that exclusively looks at MRI compliance in the obese patient, many investigators have noted that up to 30% of all patients exhibit MRI-induced anxiety or signs of claustrophobia that will frankly prevent

Table 3 Listing of potentially useful inpatient hospital needs	
Equipment	Oversized walkers Oversized bedside commodes Oversized wheelchairs Oversized or specialty beds Motorized lifting equipment Specially designated lifting teams of employees
Specialty imaging	Large-bore computed tomography scanner Bariatric magnetic resonance imaging protocol to address claustrophobia
Operating room	Tables with heavy-duty motors Radiolucent tables with higher weight limits Bariatric lines of surgical equipment and implant devices

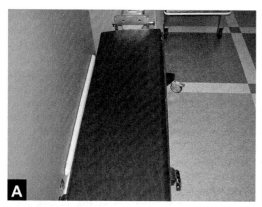
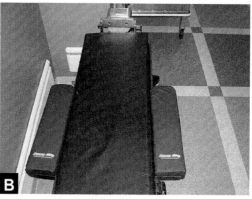

Fig. 1. Standard MizuhOSI (Mizuho OSI; Union City, CA; www.mizuhosi.com.) radiolucent operative table in use at our institution (*A*). The standard operative table width of 21.5 in can be increased by a total of 12 in with the addition of lateral arm boards (*B*). With this particular bed, several arm boards can be used per side to increase the width of the table top for its entire length.

completion of the study in up to 10% of these same patients.[49–52]

Obese individuals also present unique challenges in procedural or operating rooms. Because most medical procedures are performed on specialized tables, it should be kept in mind that the weight of a patient may exceed the weight limit of the bed in question. Again, this limit is not

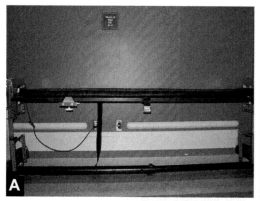
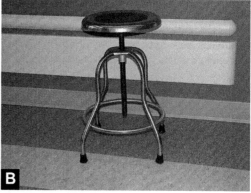
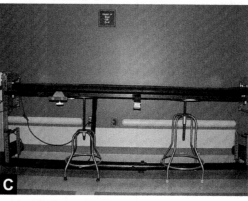

Fig. 2. Standard MizuhOSI (Mizuho OSI; Union City, CA; www.mizuhosi.com.) radiolucent operative table in use at our institution (*A*). Although thin, this table supports body weights up to 500 lb. We have increased the total weight capacity with the off-label use of standard nonrolling sitting stools (*B*) placed under the carbon composite bed with their respective seating surfaces raised to their maximum heights (*C*). The authors in no way are suggesting that readers should entertain this off-label use. It is merely being shown to illustrate the point contained in the text.

generally imposed by the risk of the bed failing to support the patient; rather, the motor responsible for fine bed movement usually imposes it. Anecdotally, there have been some ingenious solutions to the weight limit constraints including placing standard operating tables side-by-side, using arm boards attached to a standard table to help with unsupported pannus or thigh girth, and using simple sitting stools whose seating surface is raised to support the undersurface of radiolucent beds (**Figs. 1** and **2**).[53] All of these maneuvers, however, may significantly compromise or prevent mobility of the bed, the surgeon, or fluoroscopy and portable radiograph machines. Alternatively, a number of manufacturers have bariatric operative tables with motors that can accommodate up to 800 lb and table widths that can accommodate a wide variety of patient girths.[41]

Given the depth of some wounds during an invasive or an operative procedure, standard-length equipment may not allow physicians to obtain adequate access or exposure to the procedural or operative site. Again, many manufacturers of orthopedic implants and devices now have bariatric lines that offer elongated handles, offset handles that accommodate soft tissues that may be encountered within the operative field, longer retraction blades, and so forth. Readers should be prepared and willing to speak to their implant vendors, research the many devices offered, and lobby for their inclusion in lieu of or in addition to standard equipment when new capital budgets are being submitted.

SUMMARY

Prevalence rates of overweight and obesity exceed 75% for several subgroups of the US population.[7] Overweight and obese patients are necessarily becoming the norm rather than the exception in all medical practices, including orthopedic surgery. Obese individuals experience significant weight stigma and bias in the health care setting, and this bias may undermine their opportunities to receive effective medical care. Thus, a critical clinical need may lie in the areas of compassion and sensitivity toward these individuals. Orthopedic surgeons, practices, and services need to be adequately prepared to treat overweight and obese patients in a manner that allows them to feel comfortable and without stigma or stereotype. Appropriate medical devices, facilities, and staffing will be critical in the adequate assessment of an obese patient; moreover, they are essential to provide for the mental and emotional needs of these individuals in both the office and hospital environment. These should include larger blood pressure cuffs and examination gowns, durable and more accommodating furniture including examination tables, staff that have a working knowledge of the locations of items specifically suited for the obese patient, and evaluation and care plans that include an understanding of where patients must be sent if their evaluation will require a larger capacity CT or MR scanner. As the team leaders, orthopedic surgeons should ensure that as many facets of health care delivery as possible project a professional and accommodating attitude toward the overweight and obese patient.

REFERENCES

1. Flegal KM. Commentary: the epidemic of obesity—what's in a name? Int J Epidemiol 2006;35(1):72–4 [discussion: 81–2].
2. Ogden CL, Yanovski SZ, Carroll MD, et al. The epidemiology of obesity. Gastroenterology 2007; 132(6):2087–102.
3. Clinical guidelines on the identification, evaluation, and treatment of overweight and obesity in adults—the evidence report. National Institutes of Health. Obes Res 1998;6(Suppl 2):51S–209S.
4. WHO. Global strategy on diet, physical activity and health 2003. Available at: http://www.who.int/dietphysicalactivity/publications/facts/obesity/en/. Accessed April 27, 2010.
5. Ogden CL, Carroll MD, Flegal KM. Epidemiologic trends in overweight and obesity. Endocrinol Metab Clin North Am 2003;32(4):741–60, vii.
6. Flegal KM. Epidemiologic aspects of overweight and obesity in the United States. Physiol Behav 2005;86(5):599–602.
7. Flegal KM, Carroll MD, Ogden CL, et al. Prevalence and trends in obesity among US adults, 1999–2008. JAMA 2010;303(3):235–41.
8. Cdc. US obesity trends; trends by state 1985–2008. 2009. Available at: http://www.cdc.gov/obesity/data/trends.html. Accessed April 27, 2010.
9. Latner JD, O'Brien KS, Durso LE, et al. Weighing obesity stigma: the relative strength of different forms of bias. Int J Obes (Lond) 2008;32(7):1145–52.
10. Thomas SL, Hyde J, Karunaratne A, et al. Being 'fat' in today's world: a qualitative study of the lived experiences of people with obesity in Australia. Health Expect 2008;11(4):321–30.
11. Hunte HE, Williams DR. The association between perceived discrimination and obesity in a population-based multiracial and multiethnic adult sample. Am J Public Health 2009;99(7):1285–92.
12. Puhl RM, Andreyeva T, Brownell KD. Perceptions of weight discrimination: prevalence and comparison to race and gender discrimination in America. Int J Obes (Lond) 2008;32(6):992–1000.

13. Puhl RM, Brownell KD. Psychosocial origins of obesity stigma: toward changing a powerful and pervasive bias. Obes Rev 2003;4(4):213–27.

14. Andreyeva T, Puhl RM, Brownell KD. Changes in perceived weight discrimination among Americans, 1995–1996 through 2004–2006. Obesity (Silver Spring) 2008;16(5):1129–34.

15. Puhl RM, Heuer CA. Obesity stigma: important considerations for public health. Am J Public Health 2010;100(6):1019–28.

16. Puhl RM, Heuer CA. The stigma of obesity: a review and update. Obesity (Silver Spring) 2009;17(5): 941–64.

17. Brown I. Nurses' attitudes towards adult patients who are obese: literature review. J Adv Nurs 2006; 53(2):221–32.

18. Hebl MR, Xu J. Weighing the care: physicians' reactions to the size of a patient. Int J Obes Relat Metab Disord 2001;25(8):1246–52.

19. Bertakis KD, Azari R. The impact of obesity on primary care visits. Obes Res 2005;13(9):1615–23.

20. Puhl R, Brownell KD. Bias, discrimination, and obesity. Obes Res 2001;9(12):788–805.

21. Brown I, Thompson J, Tod A, et al. Primary care support for tackling obesity: a qualitative study of the perceptions of obese patients. Br J Gen Pract 2006;56(530):666–72.

22. Puhl RM, Brownell KD. Confronting and coping with weight stigma: an investigation of overweight and obese adults. Obesity (Silver Spring) 2006;14(10): 1802–15.

23. Kristeller JL, Hoerr RA. Physician attitudes toward managing obesity: differences among six specialty groups. Prev Med 1997;26(4):542–9.

24. Tarnoff M, Kaplan LM, Shikora S. An evidenced-based assessment of preoperative weight loss in bariatric surgery. Obes Surg 2008;18(9):1059–61.

25. Mrad BA, Stoklossa CJ, Birch DW. Does preoperative weight loss predict success following surgery for morbid obesity? Am J Surg 2008;195(5):570–3 [discussion: 573–4].

26. Solomon H, Liu GY, Alami R, et al. Benefits to patients choosing preoperative weight loss in gastric bypass surgery: new results of a randomized trial. J Am Coll Surg 2009;208(2):241–5.

27. Kaminsky J, Gadaleta D. A study of discrimination within the medical community as viewed by obese patients. Obes Surg 2002;12(1):14–8.

28. Lykouras L. Psychological profile of obese patients. Dig Dis 2008;26(1):36–9.

29. Whittemore AD, Kelly J, Shikora S, et al. Specialized staff and equipment for weight loss surgery patients: best practice guidelines. Obes Res 2005;13(2): 283–9.

30. Sorensen RD. A personal perspective on the needs of the weight loss surgery patient. Crit Care Nurs Q 2003;26(2):150–7.

31. Graves JW, Bailey KR, Sheps SG. The changing distribution of arm circumferences in NHANES III and NHANES 2000 and its impact on the utility of the 'standard adult' blood pressure cuff. Blood Press Monit 2003;8(6):223–7.

32. Maxwell MH, Waks AU, Schroth PC, et al. Error in blood-pressure measurement due to incorrect cuff size in obese patients. Lancet 1982;2(8288):33–6.

33. Pickering TG, Hall JE, Appel LJ, et al. Recommendations for blood pressure measurement in humans and experimental animals: part 1: blood pressure measurement in humans: a statement for professionals from the subcommittee of professional and public education of the American Heart Association Council on High Blood Pressure Research. Circulation 2005;111(5):697–716.

34. Li C, Ford ES, McGuire LC, et al. Increasing trends in waist circumference and abdominal obesity among US adults. Obesity (Silver Spring) 2007; 15(1):216–24.

35. Li C, Ford ES, Mokdad AH, et al. Recent trends in waist circumference and waist-height ratio among US children and adolescents. Pediatrics 2006;118(5):e1390–8.

36. Kramer H, Cao G, Dugas L, et al. Increasing BMI and waist circumference and prevalence of obesity among adults with type 2 diabetes: the National Health and Nutrition Examination Surveys [abstract]. J Diabet Complications 2009 [online].

37. Cooper RA. Wheelchair standards: it's all about quality assurance and evidence-based practice. J Spinal Cord Med 2006;29(2):93–4.

38. Extend-ITs. Airline coach seat sizes. 2010. Available at: http://www.extend-its.com/seatsize.htm. Accessed April 27, 2010.

39. ADA. Americans with Disabilities Act Accessibility Guidelines (ADAAG). 2004.

40. National Task Force on the Prevention and Treatment of Obesity. Medical care for obese patients: advice for health care professionals. Am Fam Physician 2002;65(1):81–8.

41. Nemarkommula AR, Singh K, Lykens K, et al. A growing market. As obesity rates rise, so do the opportunities for marketers of specialized services. Mark Health Serv 2003;23(4):34–8.

42. Buchwald H, Oien DM. Metabolic/bariatric surgery worldwide 2008. Obes Surg 2009;19(12):1605–11.

43. Davidson JE, Callery C. Care of the obesity surgery patient requiring immediate-level care or intensive care. Obes Surg 2001;11(1):93–7.

44. Pryrek KM. Caring for the obese patient. 2003. Available at: http://www.surgistrategies.com/articles/331feat2.html. Accessed April 27, 2010.

45. Pemberton V, Turner V, VanGilder C. The effect of using a low-air-loss surface on the skin integrity of obese patients: results of a pilot study. Ostomy Wound Manage 2009;55(2):44–8.

46. Compher C, Kinosian BP, Ratcliffe SJ, et al. Obesity reduces the risk of pressure ulcers in elderly hospitalized patients. J Gerontol A Biol Sci Med Sci 2007; 62(11):1310–2.

47. Philips. Brilliance CT—Big Bore Oncology. 2010. Available at: http://www.healthcare.philips.com/main/products/ct/products. Accessed April 27, 2010.

48. Siemens. SOMATOM sensation open—clinical application. 2010. Available at: http://www.medical.siemens.com/webapp/wcs/stores/servlet/. Accessed April 27, 2010.

49. McIsaac HK, Thordarson DS, Shafran R, et al. Claustrophobia and the magnetic resonance imaging procedure. J Behav Med 1998;21(3):255–68.

50. Melendez JC, McCrank E. Anxiety-related reactions associated with magnetic resonance imaging examinations. JAMA 1993;270(6):745–7.

51. Dewey M, Schink T, Dewey CF. Claustrophobia during magnetic resonance imaging: cohort study in over 55,000 patients. J Magn Reson Imaging 2007;26(5):1322–7.

52. Hollenhorst J, Munte S, Friedrich L, et al. Using intranasal midazolam spray to prevent claustrophobia induced by MR imaging. AJR Am J Roentgenol 2001;176(4):865–8.

53. Guss D, Bhattacharyya T. Perioperative management of the obese orthopaedic patient. J Am Acad Orthop Surg 2006;14(7):425–32.

Management of Upper Extremity Injuries in Obese Patients

Clifford B. Jones, MD[a,b,c],*

KEYWORDS

- Upper extremity • Obesity • Fracture • Complications

Health care costs are rising and represent 17.9% of the United States Gross Domestic Product in 2009.[1] Representing almost 10% of all medical spending in 2008, obesity is a major component of health care costs.[2] In the United States, obesity prevalence continues to increase[3–11] over the past 40 years and is associated with decreased national productivity,[12] medical expenditures,[12–15] comorbidities,[16,17] and perioperative complications.[13,18,19] Obese individuals have up to 48% greater risk of injury, incurring higher rates of trauma, and lower extremity fractures in general.[20–22] Specifically, obese people have an almost 2-fold increased chance of upper extremity injury as compared with those who are nonobese.[23] Obese patients have a higher risk of sustaining a displaced elbow fracture than normal-weight patients.[22]

This article discusses the treatment options and recommendations of upper extremity injuries in the setting of morbid obesity.

SHOULDER INJURIES

Shoulder injuries can be subgrouped into clavicular, scapular, and proximal humeral fractures. The treatment of clavicular and scapular injuries in obese patients is similar to that in nonobese patients.

Problems arise with the combination of morbid obesity and unstable displaced proximal humeral fractures. Operative treatment options for displaced proximal humeral fractures are controversial.[24,25] When combined with morbid obesity, fixation options can be problematic. A potential fixation option is closed reduction/percutaneous fixation.[26] The 2.5-mm terminally threaded Schanz pins (Synthes, Paoli, PA, USA or Zimmer, Warsaw, IN, USA) are available in 250 or 300 mm length. However, swelling associated with fracture hematoma and obesity creates arm girth wider than commercially available pin length, restricting use of this procedure until swelling abates or abandoning the procedure.

Open reduction internal fixation via a deltopectoral interval or an extended lateral deltoid-splitting approach requires a large extensile incision. Because the proximal humeral plate is applied lateral to the biceps groove, the standard deltopectoral approach can limit unobstructed plate application secondary to the muscular interval being anterior to the plate location and to the depth of the dissection. The newly modified extended anterolateral acromial approach is probably the best suited for unobstructed plate application.[27] In morbidly obese patients, the short drill sleeve and bit lengths can encumber minimally invasive plate application via submuscular plating.[28–30]

Another option for salvage of displaced unstable proximal humeral fractures is arthroplasty.[31] The problem with the deltopectoral approach and insertion of a proximal humeral arthroplasty stem is arm adduction and extension. Obesity, pendulous breasts, and wide girth all deter in line

The authors have nothing to disclose or conflicts of interest.
[a] Department of Surgery, College of Human Medicine, Michigan State University, MI, USA
[b] Van Andel Institute, 333 Bostwick Avenue NE, Grand Rapids, MI, USA
[c] Orthopaedic Associates of Michigan, 230 Michigan NE, Suite 300, Grand Rapids, MI, USA
* Orthopaedic Associates of Michigan, 230 Michigan NE, Suite 300, Grand Rapids, MI.
E-mail address: cjones@oamichigan.com

Orthop Clin N Am 42 (2011) 11–19
doi:10.1016/j.ocl.2010.08.002
0030-5898/11/$ — see front matter © 2011 Elsevier Inc. All rights reserved.

insertion of the arthroplasty stem within the humeral diaphysis. Having the patient placed onto the lateral aspect of the table with slight reverse Trendelenburg positioning can facilitate extension and adduction arm positioning. The surgeon must be prepared for all treatment methods concerning proximal humeral fixation.

Author's Preferred Method

Since utilization of the upper extremity for weight bearing or getting out of a chair is common with morbid obesity, the author prefers locking plate fixation of proximal humeral fractures to insure stable fixation, avoid pin tract infections, and enhance mobilization. For unstable, dysvascular, and nonreconstructable fractures requiring arthroplasty, the author prefers a radiolucent table in reverse with the patient in a 30° reverse Trendelenburg and in a far ipsilateral lateralized position for positioning.

HUMERAL DIAPHYSEAL INJURIES

Most of the humeral fractures can be successfully treated with closed techniques. A typical treatment algorithm is initiated with humeral realignment and reduction maintained with a coaptation splint extending from under the axilla to above the shoulder. Once swelling and pain subside, the coaptation splint is changed to a fracture or functional brace. Functional bracing relies on hydrostatic forces to maintain fracture alignment and length. Bracing is maintained until stable callus formation develops and pain diminishes. Range of motion in and out of the brace is initiated based on fracture healing and stability.

Attempts at successful closed treatment of humeral diaphyseal fractures in obese patients are fraught with problems and complications.[32,33] Splinting requires 3-point molding to achieve realignment (**Fig. 1**). With excessive adiposity, bending moments are minimal, and alignment is unable to be achieved. Furthermore, in obese women more than in men, chest wall and breast size create a varus bending moment that is unable to be counteracted with traditional closed methods. Applying a rolled towel or bump on the medial aspect of the elbow outside of the splint will potentially offset the chest wall and breast forces. Once the initial pain and swelling subside, functional bracing begins. Functional bracing requires daily utilization that increases sweating, skin breakdown, and hygiene problems. Also, with the adiposity, hydrostatic forces are diminished if not absent.[34,35] Therefore, closed methods of treating humeral diaphyseal fractures are insufficient.

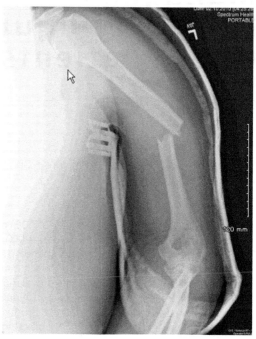

Fig. 1. Anteroposterior radiograph of failed 3-point molding of coaptation splint in the treatment of a transverse middiaphyseal humeral fracture (*arrow*).

Open treatment options in humeral diaphyseal fracture treatment are external fixation, plating, and nailing. External fixation is usually limited to temporary fixation or to situations with problematic soft tissues precluding open treatment.[36] Furthermore, neural and vascular structures limit the safe corridors for external fixation pin insertion. Because pin longevity is dependent on skin and muscle motion, adiposity increases the bone to bar distance and pin-tract irritation.

Plating of humeral fractures in obese patients should be performed in a supine or a lateral position. Prone positioning should be discouraged. Anterior approaches to the humerus should be performed for proximal or middle diaphyseal fractures, whereas posterior approaches should be performed for middle or distal diaphyseal fractures. An alternative, albeit less used, is the lateral approach, which facilitates exposure to the entire humerus but requires careful dissection around the radial neurovascular bundle. Because of the forces required for mobilization in obese patients, larger (4.5 mm not 3.5 mm, broad not narrow, and limited contact dynamic compression plates not reconstruction plates) and longer (>8 hole) plates should be applied (**Fig. 2**). Therefore, longer plates require larger exposures. Obesity and larger exposures require incisions the entire length of the humerus. Shorter incisions and smaller exposures

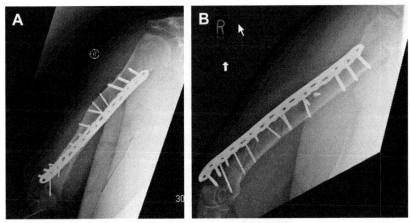

Fig. 2. Final anteroposterior (*A*) and lateral (*B*) radiographs of morbidly obese man (6 foot 5 inches, 610 pounds) with a segmental unstable middiaphyseal closed humeral fracture treated with a 16-hole 4.5-mm broad locked plate with hybrid fixation (*arrows*).

limit reduction and plate application. Also, struggling with plate application in obese settings can increase the risk of neural injury. If performed properly, humeral plating results in predictable healing with excellent alignment.[37]

Nailing of humeral fractures can be performed antegrade in a supine position or retrograde in a lateral position. Antegrade nailing is inserted through a rotator cuff incision. The arm requires adduction to assure appropriate start site positioning and trajectory. The appropriate start site and trajectory is problematic with obesity and sometimes impossible with morbid obesity. Chest wall and breast girth impedes adduction of the arm. Occasionally, extension of the arm allows enough adduction for nail insertion. Without adduction, attempted nail insertion will generate increased hoop stresses with medial wall comminution and/or varus alignment. In some cases, the lateral wall of the proximal segment can be reamed away, generating an unstable situation for nail interlock stability and increasing the risk of nonunion (**Fig. 3**). Start site entrance and proximal reaming trajectory can be enhanced with proximally inserted joysticks (2.5-mm terminally threaded Schanz pins, Synthes, Paoli, PA, USA) tilting the head into neutral or valgus and out of varus (**Fig. 4**). Furthermore, placing the patient into a bumped supine or slight lateral position with a rolled bath blanket diverts the panniculus to the contralateral flank, improves fluoroscopic visualization, and aids arm adduction (**Fig. 5**). Extreme adduction of the proximal segment with a mallet or manually with the surgeon's palm during reaming will aid anatomic alignment. It is not known if this sustained or intermittent pressure can cause radial nerve injury or not.

Lateral positioning and retrograde nail insertion through the intercondylar notch is also an option.[38–40]

Author's Preferred Method

Because morbidly obese patients require upper extremity strength and weight bearing for mobilization from a chair or with an ambulatory assistive device, the author prefers lateral positioning to minimize anesthetic risks; posterior approach to the humerus; and plating for stabilization to provide rigid, absolute stability, and early mobilization.

ELBOW INJURIES

Elbow injuries, such as olecranon, radial head, and supracondylar humeral fractures, in obese and nonobese patients are treated in a similar way. The only difference is initial splinting and treatment of elbow dislocations. Obesity negatively affects large joint dislocations.[41,42] For elbow dislocations in obese patients, problems occur with the inability to completely diagnose the injury pattern, interposing chondral fragments, and subtle joint incongruity in conjunction with poor soft tissue control with external methods.[43,44] If the elbow reduction cannot be controlled with closed methods, early diagnosis of missed chondral injuries and aggressive operative repair of ligamentous structures are paramount. The dissection is begun posterolaterally through the radiocapitellar interval. Again, because dissection planes are skewed as a result of superficial adiposity, the exposure to the radiocapitellar joint for radial head/neck fractures, capitellar fractures, and ligament reconstructions is potentially problematic. Improper dissection,

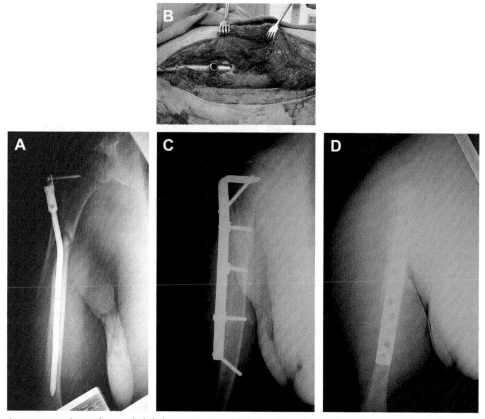

Fig. 3. Anteroposterior radiograph (*A*) demonstrates a failed nailing (varus, lateral start site) of a humeral diaphyseal fracture resulting in a painful nonunion in a morbidly obese diabetic woman. Intraoperative approach (*B*) demonstrates complete failure of the nail to capture the proximal humeral medullary canal or cortex. The nail was removed, and the nonunion was revised with a modified blade plate constructed from a 20-hole 4.5-mm broad plate. Final anteroposterior (*C*) and lateral (*D*) radiographs demonstrate realignment, bony apposition, and osseous union.

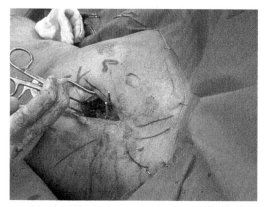

Fig. 4. Joystick insertion to the proximal humerus (2.5-mm terminally threaded Schanz pins) can rotate the head out of varus and in combination with adduction of the arm, can facilitate proper antegrade humeral nail start site location.

more extensive dissection, and supinated forearm positioning increase the risk to posterior interosseous nerve injury. Ligamentous repair and fracture reconstruction can be protected with supplemental-hinged external fixation.[45,46]

Author's Preferred Method

Within a 3- to 5-day window, the author prefers early and definitive repair of osseous and ligamentous injuries to provide stable fixation and early range of motion and to avoid supplemental bracing or external fixation.

FOREARM INJURIES

No specific issues related to obesity are noted with forearm fractures. Dissection planes can be obscured secondary to a thick adipose layer. Once reaching the fascial plane, the proper dissection plane has to be confirmed. Because adiposity and longer plate constructs mandate

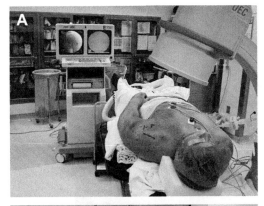

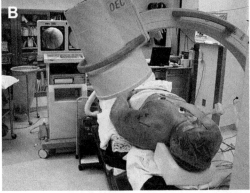

Fig. 5. Intraoperative positioning for humeral nailing with a radiolucent rolled bath blanket under the flank facilitates Grashey/anteroposterior (*A*) and Scapular Y/Lateral (*B*) visualizations of the proximal humerus and humeral diaphysis. Note that the semi-rolled position allows for slight arm extension which facilitates arm adduction.

larger exposures, incision length may approximate the entire forearm length. Once fixation is completed, check forearm supination and pronation for restoration of forearm motion and radial-ulnar stability. Close incisions over a drain to reduce potential postoperative fluid collection.

WRIST INJURIES

Most of the distal radius fractures can be successfully treated with nonoperative methods. Closed reduction and splinting can maintain fracture alignment and length.[47] Unstable fractures and morbid obesity together create a problematic combination of osseous instability and inability to create 3-point molding required for successful nonoperative management (**Fig. 6**). If closed methods fail to maintain the reduction, options for fixation are pinning, external fixation, and open reduction internal fixation. When choosing a method of operative fixation, obese patients should use the upper extremities more than nonobese patients for

mobilization with ambulatory aids and for going from supine or sitting to standing position. Pinning and external fixation of unstable distal radius fractures are possible, but one must combat pin-site irritation about the ample soft tissues and inability of casting to support the fixation.

Open reduction internal fixation provides for stable fixation that is not dependent on external casting for support. The problem with internal fixation is the exposure.[48,49] Because obesity complicates anatomic landmark visualization, the exposure must remain in the correct soft tissue plane. If not within the flexor carpi radialis sheath, dissection too ulnar or radial increases the risk of injury to the median nerve and radial artery/superficial radial nerve. Once within the correct soft tissue plane, dissection under the pronator quadratus and fixation with plates are noncomplicated. Fixation should be stable; therefore, locked volar plate fixation is recommended.[50–52]

Author's Preferred Method

The author prefers early stable volar locked plate fixation of distal radius fractures with or without ulnar styloid/shaft fixation to avoid external support or limited mobility.

ANESTHESIA FOR OBESE PATIENTS

Regional anesthetics in isolation or in combination with general anesthesia are desired for pain management in morbidly obese patients with upper extremity injuries requiring operative fixation.[53,54] Regional anesthesia can be used successfully for all upper extremity approaches except posterior Judet approaches. Mobile sonography devices may be helpful in locating specific anatomic landmarks for placement of regional anesthetic. In patients with a body mass index greater than 40, preoperative anesthesia screening is beneficial. Screening can potentially prevent or diminish obesity-related postoperative problems, such as obstructive sleep apnea, difficult airway, and gastroesophageal reflux. Regional anesthesia can reduce postoperative pain, narcotic requirements, and immobility.

Author's Preferred Method

With morbid obesity, the author prefers regional anesthesia with or without general anesthesia to improve mobilization, decrease perioperative narcotics, and facilitate return to function as soon as possible.

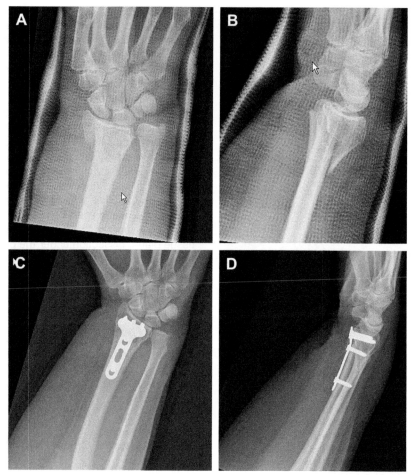

Fig. 6. Reduction anteroposterior (*A*) and lateral (*B*) radiographs with a short arm cast failing to provide any 3-point molding of a potentially unstable extraarticular distal radius fracture in a morbidly obese woman. The fracture was salvaged with a volar locked distal radius plate demonstrating the final healing with anteroposterior (*C*) and lateral (*D*) radiographs.

POSITIONING FOR OBESE PATIENTS

Because of obesity, certain operative tables are unable to withstand the weight and positioning of morbidly obese patients. If the patient is heavier (usually 500 pounds) than tolerable radiolucent limits of operative tables, certain procedures that are dependent on fluoroscopy may be limited or impossible. For example, supine antegrade humeral nailing requires a radiolucent table for localizing the starting point, fracture reduction, and distal interlocking. Therefore, humeral fractures in morbidly obese patients are more efficiently treated with plating instead of nailing.

Supine positioning and lateral positioning are favored over prone positioning in obesity.[55–58] Supine positioning is the best because of familiarity of staff and no further intraoperative positioning. However, supine positioning limits posterior approaches for humeral retrograde nailing and intercondylar humeral fixation. Lateral positioning requires many staff to safely lift and rotate these patients to avoid injury to staff and the patient (**Fig. 7**). Some patients require clamped body restrains to assist the beanbag positioner because of patients' width and overwhelming weight. Because of the width of some obese patients, step stools are required for surgeon visualization. Prone positioning is the most problematic and should be avoided. Complications such as inability to ventilate the patient, facial and orbital injury, brachial plexus injury, and paralysis have been noted.[58–61]

Author's Preferred Method

With morbid obesity, the author prefers lateral or supine (in slight reverse Trendelenburg) positioning for fixation of upper extremity fractures.

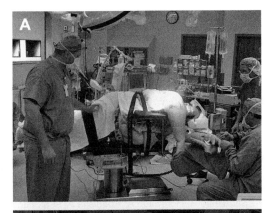

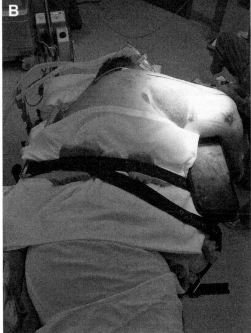

Fig. 7. Intraoperative positioning (*A, B*) of a 6 ft 5 in tall and 610 pound, 35–year-old man with a closed segmental humeral fracture that failed conservative management with coaptation splinting and functional bracing. Note the lateral positioning on an industrial strength table, beanbag support, many staff to assist, padding of all safety straps, and sequential compression devices on the lower extremities.

SUMMARY

Obesity is a big problem concerning orthopedic injuries and treatment. Obesity increases the risk of upper extremity injury when falling. Splinting or casting is problematic and ineffectual for management of upper extremity injuries in obese patients. Regional anesthesia, which is capable of providing upper extremity perioperative pain relief, is favored over general anesthesia secondary to reducing

narcotic use, obstructive sleep apnea, obstructive airway disease, and gastroesophageal reflux. Lateral and supine positionings are less problematic than prone positioning. Some upper extremity procedures are problematic if not impossible with positioning, body habitus, and exposure limitations with obesity. Stable operative fixation produces predictable results with upper extremity fractures in obese patients.

REFERENCES

1. Sisko A, Truffer C, Smith S, et al. Health spending projections through 2018: recession effects add uncertainty to the outlook. Health Aff (Millwood) 2009;28(2):w346–57.
2. Finkelstein EA, Fiebelkorn IC, Wang G. State-level estimates of annual medical expenditures attributable to obesity. Obes Res 2004;12(1):18–24.
3. Ogden CL, Troiano RP, Briefel RR, et al. Prevalence of overweight among preschool children in the United States, 1971 through 1994. Pediatrics 1997; 99(4):E1.
4. Flegal KM, Carroll MD, Kuczmarski RJ, et al. Overweight and obesity in the United States: prevalence and trends, 1960–1994. Int J Obes Relat Metab Disord 1998;22(1):39–47.
5. Flegal KM, Carroll MD, Ogden CL, et al. Prevalence and trends in obesity among US adults, 1999–2000. JAMA 2002;288(14):1723–7.
6. Flegal KM, Troiano RP. Changes in the distribution of body mass index of adults and children in the US population. Int J Obes Relat Metab Disord 2000; 24(7):807–18.
7. Harlan WR, Landis JR, Flegal KM, et al. Secular trends in body mass in the United States, 1960–1980. Am J Epidemiol 1988;128(5):1065–74.
8. Kuczmarski RJ, Flegal KM, Campbell SM, et al. Increasing prevalence of overweight among US adults. The National Health and Nutrition Examination Surveys, 1960 to 1991. JAMA 1994;272(3): 205–11.
9. Mokdad AH, Ford ES, Bowman BA, et al. Prevalence of obesity, diabetes, and obesity-related health risk factors, 2001. JAMA 2003;289(1):76–9.
10. Ogden CL, Carroll MD, Curtin LR, et al. Prevalence of overweight and obesity in the United States, 1999–2004. JAMA 2006;295(13):1549–55.
11. Troiano RP, Flegal KM, Kuczmarski RJ, et al. Overweight prevalence and trends for children and adolescents. The National Health and Nutrition Examination Surveys, 1963 to 1991. Arch Pediatr Adolesc Med 1995;149(10):1085–91.
12. Finkelstein E, Fiebelkorn C, Wang G. The costs of obesity among full-time employees. Am J Health Promot 2005;20(1):45–51.

13. Flancbaum L, Choban PS. Surgical implications of obesity. Annu Rev Med 1998;49:215–34.
14. Finkelstein EA, Fiebelkorn IC, Wang G. National medical spending attributable to overweight and obesity: how much, and who's paying? Health Aff (Millwood) 2003;(Suppl Web Exclusives): W3-219–W3-26.
15. Arterburn DE, Maciejewski ML, Tsevat J. Impact of morbid obesity on medical expenditures in adults. Int J Obes (Lond) 2005;29(3):334–9.
16. Must A, Spadano J, Coakley EH, et al. The disease burden associated with overweight and obesity. JAMA 1999;282(16):1523–9.
17. Pi-Sunyer FX. Medical hazards of obesity. Ann Intern Med 1993;119(7 Pt 2):655–60.
18. Dindo D, Muller MK, Weber M, et al. Obesity in general elective surgery. Lancet 2003;361(9374): 2032–5.
19. Choban PS, Heckler R, Burge JC, et al. Increased incidence of nosocomial infections in obese surgical patients. Am Surg 1995;61(11):1001–5.
20. Meroz Y, Gozal Y. Management of the obese trauma patient. Anesthesiol Clin 2007;25(1):91–8, ix.
21. Finkelstein EA, Chen H, Prabhu M, et al. The relationship between obesity and injuries among U.S. adults. Am J Health Promot 2007;21(5):460–8.
22. Bostman OM. Body mass index of patients with elbow and ankle fractures requiring surgical treatment. J Trauma 1994;37(1):62–5.
23. Davidson PL, Goulding A, Chalmers DJ. Biomechanical analysis of arm fracture in obese boys. J Paediatr Child Health 2003;39(9):657–64.
24. Court-Brown CM, Cattermole H, McQueen MM. Impacted valgus fractures (B1.1) of the proximal humerus. The results of non-operative treatment. J Bone Joint Surg Br 2002;84(4):504–8.
25. Court-Brown CM, Garg A, McQueen MM. The translated two-part fracture of the proximal humerus. Epidemiology and outcome in the older patient. J Bone Joint Surg 2001;83(6):799–804.
26. Jaberg H, Warner JJ, Jakob RP. Percutaneous stabilization of unstable fractures of the humerus. J Bone Joint Surg Am 1992;74(4):508–15.
27. Gardner MJ, Griffith MH, Dines JS, et al. The extended anterolateral acromial approach allows minimally invasive access to the proximal humerus. Clin Orthop Relat Res 2005;434:123–9.
28. Gardner MJ, Griffith MH, Dines JS, et al. A minimally invasive approach for plate fixation of the proximal humerus. Bull Hosp Jt Dis 2004; 62(1–2):18–23.
29. Rouleau DM, Laflamme GY, Berry GK, et al. Proximal humerus fractures treated by percutaneous locking plate internal fixation. Orthop Traumatol Surg Res 2009;95(1):56–62.
30. Laflamme GY, Rouleau DM, Berry GK, et al. Percutaneous humeral plating of fractures of the proximal humerus: results of a prospective multicenter clinical trial. J Orthop Trauma 2008;22(3):153–8.
31. Fialka C, Stampfl P, Arbes S, et al. Primary hemiarthroplasty in four-part fractures of the proximal humerus: randomized trial of two different implant systems. J Shoulder Elbow Surg 2008;17(2):210–5.
32. Jawa A, McCarty P, Doornberg J, et al. Extra-articular distal-third diaphyseal fractures of the humerus. A comparison of functional bracing and plate fixation. J Bone Joint Surg Am 2006;88(11):2343–7.
33. Rutgers M, Ring D. Treatment of diaphyseal fractures of the humerus using a functional brace. J Orthop Trauma 2006;20(9):597–601.
34. Sarmiento A, Horowitch A, Aboulafia A, et al. Functional bracing for comminuted extra-articular fractures of the distal third of the humerus. J Bone Joint Surg 1990;72(2):283–7.
35. Sarmiento A, Kinman PB, Galvin EG, et al. Functional bracing of fractures of the shaft of the humerus. J Bone Joint Surg Am 1977;59(5):596–601.
36. Marsh JL, Mahoney CR, Steinbronn D. External fixation of open humerus fractures. Iowa Orthop J 1999; 19:35–42.
37. Chapman JR, Henley MB, Agel J, et al. Randomized prospective study of humeral shaft fracture fixation: intramedullary nails versus plates. J Orthop Trauma 2000;14(3):162–6.
38. Stannard JP, Harris HW, McGwin G Jr, et al. Intramedullary nailing of humeral shaft fractures with a locking flexible nail. J Bone Joint Surg Am 2003;85(11): 2103–10.
39. Halder SC, Chapman JA, Choudhury G, et al. Retrograde fixation of fractures of the neck and shaft of the humerus with the 'Halder humeral nail'. Injury 2001;32(9):695–703.
40. Blum J, Janzing H, Gahr R, et al. Clinical performance of a new medullary humeral nail: antegrade versus retrograde insertion. J Orthop Trauma 2001; 15(5):342–9.
41. Peltola EK, Lindahl J, Hietaranta H, et al. Knee dislocation in overweight patients. AJR Am J Roentgenol 2009;192(1):101–6.
42. Marin EL, Bifulco SS, Fast A. Obesity. A risk factor for knee dislocation. Am J Phys Med Rehabil 1990; 69(3):132–4.
43. Saati AZ, McKee MD. Fracture-dislocation of the elbow: diagnosis, treatment, and prognosis. Hand Clin 2004;20(4):405–14.
44. Ring D, Hannouche D, Jupiter JB. Surgical treatment of persistent dislocation or subluxation of the ulnohumeral joint after fracture-dislocation of the elbow. J Hand Surg Am 2004;29(3):470–80.
45. Ruch DS, Triepel CR. Hinged elbow fixation for recurrent instability following fracture dislocation. Injury 2001;32(Suppl 4):SD70–8.
46. Zilkens C, Graf M, Anastasiadis A, et al. Treatment of acute and chronic elbow instability with a hinged

external fixator after fracture dislocation. Acta Orthop Belg 2009;75(2):167–74.

47. Fernandez DL. Closed manipulation and casting of distal radius fractures. Hand Clin 2005;21(3):307–16.

48. Orbay J, Badia A, Khoury RK, et al. Volar fixed-angle fixation of distal radius fractures: the DVR plate. Tech Hand Up Extrem Surg 2004;8(3):142–8.

49. Orbay JL, Badia A, Indriago IR, et al. The extended flexor carpi radialis approach: a new perspective for the distal radius fracture. Tech Hand Up Extrem Surg 2001;5(4):204–11.

50. Drobetz H, Bryant AL, Pokorny T, et al. Volar fixed-angle plating of distal radius extension fractures: influence of plate position on secondary loss of reduction—a biomechanic study in a cadaveric model. J Hand Surg Am 2006;31(4):615–22.

51. Elsaidi GA, Deal N, Smith BP, et al. Volar collapse after dorsal plating of comminuted distal radius fractures. Am J Orthop 2007;36(5):269–72.

52. Gruber G, Gruber K, Giessauf C, et al. Volar plate fixation of AO type C2 and C3 distal radius fractures, a single-center study of 55 patients. J Orthop Trauma 2008;22(7):467–72.

53. Chung SA, Yuan H, Chung F. A systemic review of obstructive sleep apnea and its implications for anesthesiologists. Anesth Analg 2008;107(5): 1543–63.

54. Isono S. Obstructive sleep apnea of obese adults: pathophysiology and perioperative airway management. Anesthesiology 2009;110(4):908–21.

55. Swerdlow BN, Brodsky JB, Butcher MD. Placement of a morbidly obese patient in the prone position. Anesthesiology 1988;68(4):657–8.

56. Bentley JB, Vaughan RW. Prone positioning in obesity. Anesth Analg 1981;60(7):537.

57. Porter SE, Graves ML, Qin Z, et al. Operative experience of pelvic fractures in the obese. Obes Surg 2008;18(6):702–8.

58. Goettler CE, Pryor JP, Reilly PM. Brachial plexopathy after prone positioning. Crit Care 2002;6(6):540–2.

59. Schwartz H. Problems of obesity in anesthesia. N Y State J Med 1955;55(22):3277–81.

60. Feinberg GL. Obesity: class IV anesthesia risk. N Y State J Med 1971;71(8):2200–1.

61. Brodsky JB. Positioning the morbidly obese patient for anesthesia. Obes Surg 2002;12(6):751–8.

Management of Femur Shaft Fractures in Obese Patients

Philipp N. Streubel, MD*, Michael J. Gardner, MD,
William M. Ricci, MD

KEYWORDS

- Femur fracture • Obesity • Intramedullary nailing
- Outcomes

Given the ongoing epidemic of obesity, femoral fracture management in the population affected by this condition is likely to become more frequent. Obesity in the United States has been steadily increasing over the last few decades, rising from 13.3% in 1960 to 31% in 2002.[1] Similarly, the prevalence of obesity has dramatically increased among children from 10 to 17 years from 6% in 2003 to 16% in 2007. Also, obesity increased by up to 33% among Hispanic children and children from single-parent households,[2] with rates reported as high as 40%.[3,4] Extreme obesity (body mass index [BMI] >40 kg/m^2) has further increased from 2.9% from 1988 to 1994 to 4.7% from 1999 to 2000,[5] and was reported to be 5.7% from 2007 to 2008 with an especially high prevalence in non-Hispanic black women (14.2%).[6]

Fracture treatment in obese patients poses a special challenge, given the greater difficulty in establishing an accurate diagnosis and confirming associated injuries. Adequate intraoperative positioning and obtaining accurate reduction and stable fixation may require special considerations. Obese patients have a high predisposition for complications such as compartment syndrome, nerve injuries, and pressure ulcers, and are at increased risk for medical complications given the high prevalence of comorbidities.[7–11] A thorough understanding of the risks associated with obesity and the diagnostic and therapeutic challenges involved with femoral shaft fractures in this setting is paramount to achieve adequate results.

THE OBESE PATIENT

Obese patients have lower self-reported health-related quality of life[12] as well as an increased risk of having coronary artery disease, type 2 diabetes mellitus, and endometrial, breast, colon cancer, hypertension, dyslipidemia, stroke, gallbladder disease, osteoarthritis, sleep apnea, and respiratory problems.[8] As a consequence, obese patients carry an increased risk for systemic complications including infection, deep venous thrombosis, myocardial infarction, and pneumonia.[10,11,13,14] Maheshwari and colleagues[9] studied the effect of obesity on the morbidity of patients who suffered femur or tibia fractures during a motor vehicle collision. In a cohort of 665 patients, obese subjects had a higher prevalence of reported baseline cardiac disease and diabetes compared with non-obese patients. Furthermore, obese patients had more severe fracture patterns involving the distal femur (90% vs 61%, $P<.01$). No differences were found in postoperative complications, but obese patients had an almost 2-fold mortality risk that approached statistical significance (9.5% vs 5.6%, $P = .07$). Other studies on critically injured blunt trauma patients have confirmed obesity as an independent risk factor for mortality, increased hospital and intensive care unit length of stay, and prolonged use of mechanical ventilation in

Orthopaedic Trauma Service, Department of Orthopaedic Surgery, Washington University School of Medicine, 660 South Euclid Avenue, Campus Box 8233 St Louis, MO 63110, USA
* Corresponding author.
E-mail address: philipp.streubel@gmail.com

Orthop Clin N Am 42 (2011) 21–35
doi:10.1016/j.ocl.2010.07.004

survivors.[15–17] Regarding nosocomial infections, Choban and colleagues[14] compared a cohort of 849 patients undergoing general, urologic, vascular, thoracic, or gynecologic surgical procedures and found an increased incidence in patients with higher BMI. Although infections occurred in 0.5% of patients with BMI of less than 27 kg/m^2, frequencies increased to 2.8% in patients with BMI of 27 to 31 kg/m^2 and 4.3% in patients with BMI greater than 31 kg/m^2. Wound healing problems have additionally been found to be more frequent in obese patients undergoing acetabular and femoral fracture fixation, with diabetes and the presence of extensive panniculus contributing to the occurrence of this complication.[11,13]

INCIDENCE AND MECHANISM OF INJURY

Despite femoral shaft fractures having been a subject of extensive research, only limited literature has focused on the management of these fractures in the obese population. According to Tucker and colleagues,[18] 20% of patients with femur fractures are obese (BMI ≥30 kg/m^2), with an obesity rate among women of 32% compared with 15% in men. Motor vehicle accidents account for about 50% of femoral shaft fractures. This proportion is similar between obese and nonobese individuals. Sports and motorcycle accidents account for a substantial proportion of fractures in nonobese patients but not in obese patients, presumably because the latter are less frequently engaged in these activities. Falls, however, account for 31% of femur fractures in obese patients compared with only 14% in nonobese individuals.[18] Furthermore, it is not infrequent in obese individuals for fractures to occur unrelated to or after only a minimal traumatic event. Although the absence of significant trauma may lead to the perception of the fracture having been caused by low energy, the opposite is, however, most likely the case. Contrary to nonobese patients in whom low-velocity fractures are likely to be related to decreased bone mineral density, in obese individuals they occur in the presence of increased bone mineral density and bone cross-section area.[19] Owing to a large body mass, even at low trauma velocities, significant energy can be generated leading to significant fracture comminution and soft-tissue damage.[9]

DIAGNOSIS

Heightened suspicion for a femoral fracture should be present in the obese patient with marked thigh pain after even minor trauma. Given the large body habitus, fractures of the femur may not be readily apparent in the patient population. Concomitant injuries to ipsilateral and contralateral acetabulum, pelvis, hip, and knee should be actively ruled out during the secondary survey, as the probability of these going unnoticed is increased in the patient population.[20] Dedicated views for the hip and knee as well as trauma series for pelvis and acetabulum should be taken. In the general population up to 9% of femoral shaft fractures have an associated femoral neck fracture, of which up to 50% are missed at initial assessment (**Fig. 1**).[21–23] Although no specific data have been published for obese patients, this population is at increased risk for missed diagnosis owing to poor visualization of the femoral neck given the presence of large amounts of adipose tissue. Although active screening for these fractures on femur radiographs as well as specific internal rotation hip views should be performed, computed tomography scans of the proximal femur may be indicated in this patient population.[21,23,24] In a cohort of 152 femoral shaft fractures, Yang and colleagues[23] found 12 femoral neck fractures at the moment of admission. Of these, a total of 6 nondisplaced fractures were not detectable using conventional radiography but could be observed on computed tomography (CT) scans. Tornetta and colleagues[21] showed that fine-cut (2 mm) CT scanning of the proximal femur was able to detect 12 of 13 (92%) femoral neck fractures associated with fractures of the ipsilateral femoral shaft, as opposed to only 8 (62%) fractures using only hip radiographs. Furthermore, with CT scanning the incidence of delayed diagnosis could be reduced from 57% to 6%, allowing for earlier femoral neck fracture recognition and management. CT scanning is of additional use for the postoperative assessment of the acetabulum and femoral neck after closed reduction of associated ipsilateral hip dislocations (**Fig. 2**).

Obese patients are at higher risk of having comminuted fractures. According to Tucker and colleagues,[18] whereas nonobese patients had comminuted (Orthopedic Trauma Association type C) fractures in 18% of cases, obese patients had comminution in 25% of cases. Open fractures occurred with equal frequency in obese and nonobese patients in 17% and 16% of cases, respectively. However, no type III open fractures were found in obese patients, whereas they accounted for 35% of open fractures in nonobese patients. This finding may suggest that femur fractures in obese patients rarely lead to inadequate soft-tissue coverage; however, open fractures in this patient population should suggest an even higher level of energy, as expected for this type of fracture in nonobese subjects. Furthermore, a high

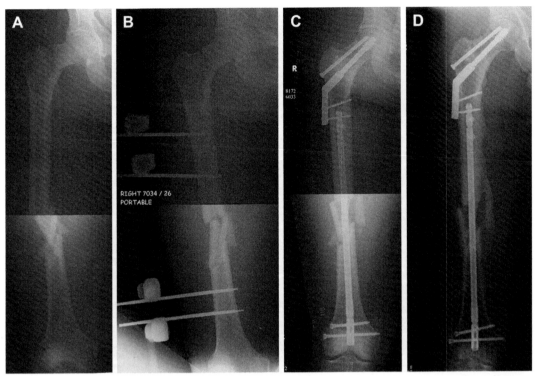

Fig. 1. A 34-year-old man (BMI 36 kg/m^2) who suffered a femoral shaft fracture and concomitant ipsilateral femoral neck fracture (*A*). Owing to physiologic instability, the patient underwent initial fracture stabilization of the shaft with a unilateral external fixator (*B*). Delayed treatment included retrograde femoral nailing of the femoral shaft, and proximal fixation with a sliding hip screw and antirotational screw (*C*). Six months after surgery, profuse fracture callus can be seen both at the femoral neck and shaft (*D*).

level of suspicion should be present regarding vascular injury, given the clinical difficulty for assessing such an injury. The ankle brachial index (ABI) is considered the test of choice for the initial assessment of vascular injury in the lower extremity. To perform this test in obese patients, however, a special cuff may be necessary that fits the increased circumference of the calf. An ABI of less than 0.9 should prompt additional vascular investigations.[25–27]

Skeletal traction using either smooth Kirschner wires with bow tensioner or threaded Steinman pins inserted from medial to lateral at the level of the superior pole of the patella may be required for initial fracture stabilization and pain management. Although traction with 15 lb (6.8 kg) is usually sufficient for nonobese patients, significantly higher weights may be required in morbidly obese patients and should be calculated at approximately 10% to 15% of body weight.[28]

PERIOPERATIVE CONSIDERATIONS

Because of increased body habitus, special surgical equipment is frequently required. Special surgical equipment includes larger and stronger

tables, special supports, as well as specially designed instruments. In a group of obese patients with a BMI ranging from 33.2 to 57.1 kg/m^2 undergoing nonunion surgery, Jupiter and colleagues[7] reported on the occurrence of several complications including peroneal compartment syndrome, gluteal compartment syndrome with sciatic nerve palsy, bilateral brachial plexus stretch injuries, anterior interosseous nerve palsy, and postoperative development of a patch of scalp alopecia. These complications were thought to be related in every case with poorly protective positioning and prolonged ischemic pressure under the patient's body weight during the surgical procedure. Therefore, adequate padding of bony prominences as well as continuous intraoperative monitoring of compartment tension of the contralateral leg and buttock should be performed.

To achieve adequate fracture visualization, image intensifiers with good imaging quality are required. Owing to the high prevalence of femoral neck fractures in the presence of femoral shaft fractures, imaging quality is of special relevance in this setting, because the large amount of soft tissue may obscure adequate visualization. Intraarticular injection of contrast medium has been

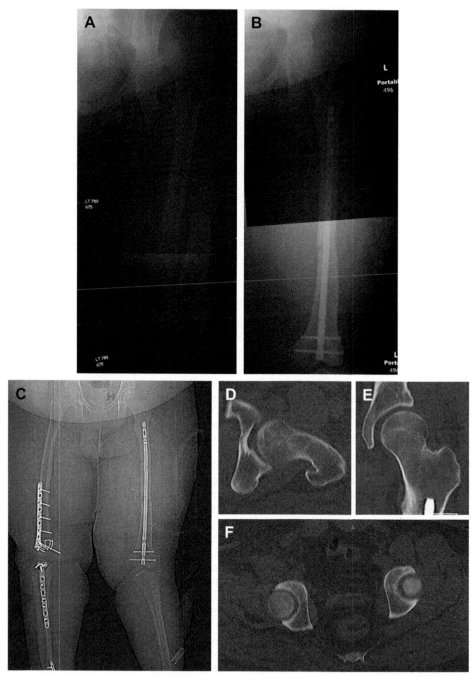

Fig. 2. An 18-year-old man (BMI 64 kg/m²) who was admitted with a left femoral shaft fracture and ipsilateral posterior hip dislocation. Other injuries included proximal and distal tibia and distal femur fractures of the contralateral lower extremity (*A*). He underwent closed hip reduction, retrograde nailing of the left femur (*B*), and open reduction internal fixation of the right femur and tibia (*C*). Femoral neck fractures were excluded with axial CT views (*D*) and coronal reconstructions of the pelvis (*E*). Axial CT view shows adequate reduction of the left hip and a marginal fracture of the posterior wall of the acetabulum (*F*).

proposed to enhance visualization of the femoral head in massively obese patients, to facilitate adequate screw placement when cephalomedullary devices are required and to rule out iatrogenic fractures of the femoral neck after intramedullary nailing.[29]

TREATMENT

Assessment and management of obese patients should be addressed in a similar fashion to nonobese patients, and should follow the guidelines of the advanced trauma life support. An important consideration in the initial physiologic stabilization of these patients is that despite the large body mass, total blood volume in obese individuals is similar to that of normal-sized individuals because excess body mass is mainly composed of adipose tissue. As a consequence, the percentage of blood loss caused by femoral fracture should be calculated in relation to lean body mass rather than total patient weight.[30]

Fracture stabilization should adjust to the patient's physiologic reserve, with early definitive fracture fixation in the stable patient and temporary stabilization after damage-control guidelines in unstable individuals with additional major injuries (**Fig. 3**). Given the increased rate of complications and the prolonged metabolic acidosis of obese patients, even after adequate resuscitation, a lower threshold for a damage-control approach should exist.[30] Similar to nonobese patients, the presence of concomitant head and/or chest trauma may indicate initial external fixation in order to reduce the risk of acute respiratory distress syndrome and multiorgan failure.[31]

External fixation is considered the method of choice for temporary fixation in unstable patients, and can be safely followed by staged intramedullary nailing.[32,33] In morbidly obese patients, however, fixation may be challenging to achieve, given the long distance between the skin surface and the femoral cortex (**Figs. 4** and **5**).[34] Tactile feedback as well as visual orientation using an image intensifier should lead to adequate pin placement. Given the large loads the construct supports, additional pins may be required as well as the use of double bars for fracture bridging. Nonreamed retrograde nailing with or without locking has been recently proposed as an alternative to temporary external fixation.[35]

FRACTURE FIXATION

Reamed antegrade intramedullary nailing through the piriformis fossa is considered the gold standard for most diaphyseal femur fractures, with reported healing rates of 86% to 100%.[36–39] In obese patients, however, obtaining an adequate starting point at the proximal femur may be challenging, requiring long surgical procedures and large incisions (see **Fig. 5**).[18] As a consequence, increased bleeding and wound-healing complications can be expected.[10] In a retrospective study, McKee and Waddell[10] identified 7 morbidly obese patients (200% of ideal weight or ≥100 lb [45.36 kg] more than ideal body weight or BMI ≥37 kg/m^2) who underwent antegrade reamed femoral nailing over a 5-year period. Mean surgical duration was 3.8 hours and intraoperative blood loss averaged 1100 mL. Several complications occurred, including greater trochanter fractures due to difficulty obtaining starting point, wound infections, deep vein thrombosis, and fatal pulmonary embolus. When antegrade nailing is chosen, patient positioning on a fracture table with skeletal traction and the well leg abducted and in hemilithotomy may be indicated. Elevated calf compartment pressure in this position may, however, increase the risk for compartment syndrome and should therefore be carefully monitored.[40] Although scissoring the legs may be appropriate positioning in nonobese patients, it may not be feasible in obese patients. Traction may be obtained using a boot; skeletal traction may, however, provide increased control of fracture alignment. In more proximal fractures, placing the perineal post on the contralateral ischium allows for improved adduction of the proximal fragment. Lateral tilting of the patient may improve access to the proximal femur by allowing an abdominal panniculus to fall away from the surgical field (see **Fig. 5**). For very large patients, a fracture table may not be sturdy enough to support the patient. In such a setting, the patient may be placed on a radiolucent flat-top table for a free leg antegrade femoral nailing. Skeletal traction may be applied to the operative limb by using an attachment to the end of the table from which to suspend the weights.

In addition, trochanteric entry nails should be considered in this setting. In a series of 12 fractures and 3 nonunions of the femoral shaft treated with antegrade trochanteric entry nails in 14 patients who were either overweight, obese, or had trochanteric lypodystrophy, Ostrum[41] obtained adequate healing in 12 cases. Of the 3 resulting nonunions, 2 were associated with hardware failure. Furthermore, 1 patient had a transient pudendal nerve palsy. Based on these results, the tip of the trochanter may be the access of choice when antegrade femoral nailing is required in obese patients.

Given the lower amount of soft tissue present around the knee, retrograde nailing has become

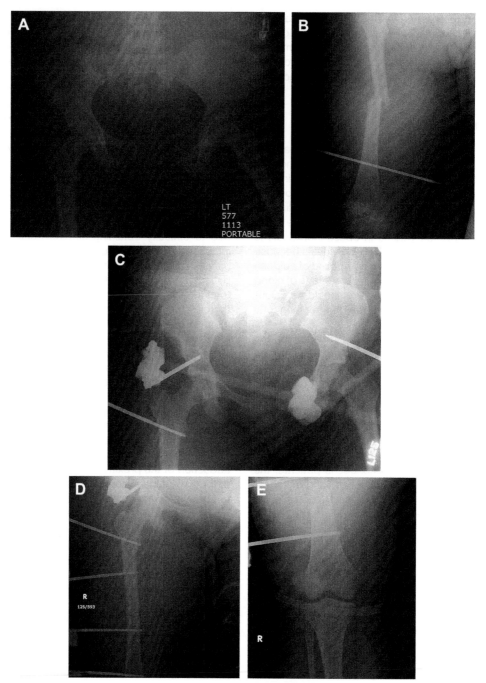

Fig. 3. An 18-year-old woman (BMI 46 kg/m^2) who was struck by a motor vehicle, suffering closed head injury, bilateral vertically unstable pelvic injuries (*A*), and a right femoral shaft fracture with vascular injury (*B*). Management included skeletal traction and external fixation of the pelvis (*C*) and femur (*D*, *E*). Distal above-the-knee amputation was required owing to dysvascular distal lower extremity. The patient died of traumatic brain injury.

the treatment of choice in morbidly obese patients (**Fig. 6**). Tucker and colleagues[18] compared the outcomes of intramedullary nailing of femoral shaft fractures in obese (BMI ≥30 kg/m^2) and nonobese patients (BMI <30 kg/m^2) using either antegrade or retrograde nails. Antegrade nailing was on average 30 minutes longer in obese than in nonobese patients (94 vs 62 minutes, respectively) and required significantly longer irradiation (247 vs 135 seconds, respectively). No differences were

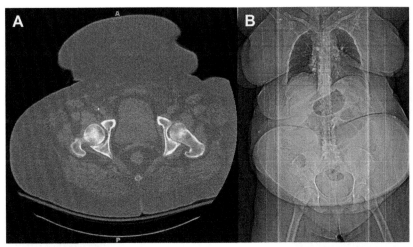

Fig. 4. Axial cut (*A*) and anteroposterior scout view of a morbidly obese subject (BMI 60 kg/m^2) (*B*). Note the marked distance between the proximal femur and the cutaneous surface.

found among groups when retrograde nailing was performed. More importantly, in the obese group retrograde nailing was performed in a significantly shorter time with less irradiation than antegrade nailing (94 vs 67 minutes and 242 vs 76 seconds, respectively). Although no significant differences in healing rate and final functional recovery based on the lower extremity measure were observed, obese patients were found to recover at a slower rate and to a lesser extent than patients who were not obese. Some investigators have reported higher rates of rotational and coronal malalignment as well as shortening using retrograde nailing.[42] Similar healing and malunion rates after either retrograde or antegrade nailing of femoral shaft fractures have, however, also been reported.[43] Knee pain has been reported as a prevalent problem after retrograde nailing; similar rates of hip pain can, however, be expected for antegrade nailing.[43] While obesity has become an indication for retrograde nailing, several other circumstances further increase the appropriateness for this fixation technique, including polytrauma, bilateral femur fractures, acetabular injuries, floating knee fractures, pregnancy, and ipsilateral femoral neck fractures **Fig. 7**.[22,39,44–52] summarizes the surgical technique for retrograde nailing.

Retrograde nailing of the femur, however, requires the fracture to be located at least 5 cm distal to the lesser trochanter, and is therefore considered contraindicated in proximal subtrochanteric fractures. In extremely large patients an adequate proximal starting point may not be achievable, and proximal fixation may be obtained by advancing a retrograde guide wire through the proximal femoral cortex into the piriformis fossa, with subsequent reaming and nail insertion (**Fig. 8**).

When treating femoral shaft fractures in obese patients, construct strength should be maximized. Not only does the increased body mass subject the implant to higher loads, but obese patients are also frequently less likely to be compliant with no or partial weight bearing because of their limitations in mobility. Reamed nailing allows for a more stable construct in several ways. For isthmic fractures, reamed nailing increases cortical contact area between the endosteum and the nail. Furthermore, reaming allows the insertion of increased diameter nails. Because the torsional and bending strengths of a cylinder are proportional to the fourth and third power of the radius, respectively, small increases in nail diameter can have a significant effect on construct strength. However, overeager reaming of the medullary canal may lead to excessive vascular damage, heat necrosis, and subsequent impairment of the local anatomy.[53,54] Reaming until initial cortical chatter is heard and felt should, therefore, lead to adequate canal preparation.

Whereas in nonobese patients axially stable fractures (Winquist 1 and 2) can be safely managed with intramedullary nails in dynamic interlocking mode,[38] in obese patients a low threshold for static locking as well as the use of multiple-locking screws should be present. Due to increased patient weight secondary cortical comminution may more frequently occur, thereby leading to loss of axial stability. Furthermore, in retrograde nailing, distal interlock breakage leads to distal telescoping of the nail and subsequent knee-joint injury, and therefore requires distal

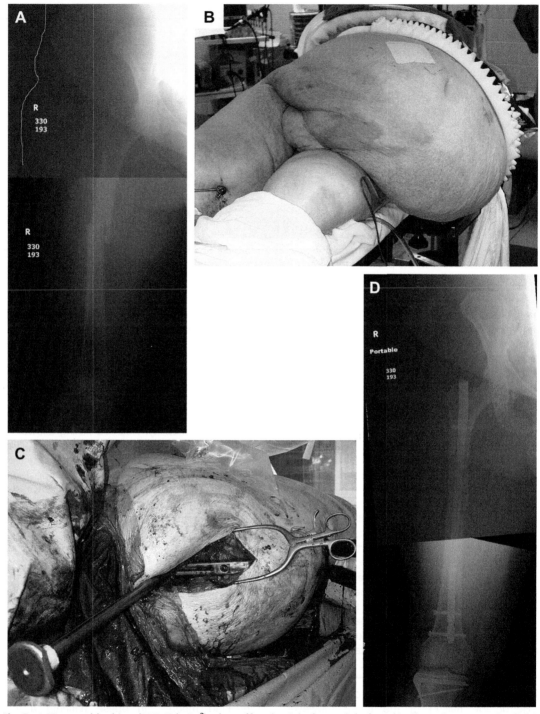

Fig. 5. A 55-year-old subject (BMI 42 kg/m²) who suffered a right femoral shaft and ipsilateral open proximal tibia fracture during a motor vehicle accident. Note the distance between the cutaneous surface (*white line*) and the proximal femur (*A*). Slight lateral positioning aided in clearing the surgical site from prominent adipose tissue (*B*). Femoral shaft fracture fixation was performed with an antegrade intramedullary nail. The patient's large body habitus made a large skin incision necessary to obtain an adequate starting point. Furthermore, note that the distance of the vertical arm of the insertion handle of the nail and the femur is not sufficient to clear the patient's soft tissues. By creating a tunnel through the lateral adipose tissue, proximal locking could be performed through small stab incisions in the skin of the lateral thigh under fluoroscopic guidance (*C*). Postoperative result shows reduction and fixation of both the femoral shaft and proximal tibia (*D*).

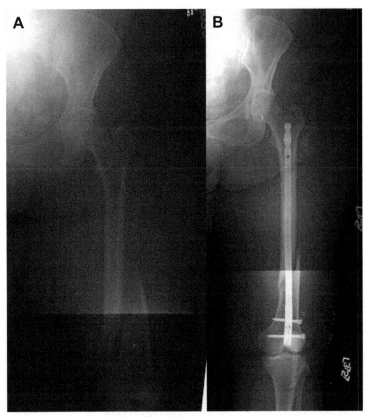

Fig. 6. A 72-year-old patient (BMI 32 kg/m²) who suffered a spiral femoral shaft fracture after a fall (*A*). Postoperative result after retrograde intramedullary nailing (*B*).

interlocking to occur with at least 2 screws.[55] Using a biomechanical comminuted fracture model, Brumback and colleagues[56] showed that antegrade 12-mm nails with 2 distal interlocking screws were significantly stronger than those with only 1 interlocking screw. Furthermore, adequate fracture reduction was maintained and healing obtained in a series of 28 comminuted femur fractures treated with a 12-mm Russell Taylor nail (Smith and Nephew, Memphis, TN) with 2 distal interlocking screws. Immediate postoperative weight bearing was allowed in all patients. The average patient weight was 81 kg (range 50–127 kg).

IPSILATERAL FEMORAL NECK FRACTURES

As much as 10% of patients with femur fractures can present with an ipsilateral femoral neck fracture.[21–23] Although several modalities, including antegrade nailing with cannulated miss-a-nail screw technique, cephalomedullary nailing, and retrograde nailing with cannulated or sliding hip screw fixation, have been proposed for management in the general population, retrograde

nailing is probably the most indicated in the obese population. As discussed, retrograde nailing has clear advantages over antegrade nailing for the management of femoral shaft fractures in this patient population. Furthermore, it allows the use of a proximal sliding hip screw, which may be the implant of choice for proximal fixation in these patients given its improved strength compared with cannulated screws.[57] Moreover, in combination with an antirotational screw, sliding hip screws are the implant of choice for subcapital vertical shear fractures that are frequently found in this setting (see **Fig. 1**).[58–61]

OPEN FRACTURES

Given the large soft-tissue envelope, open femur fractures are rare in obese patients. If open femur fractures occur, however, a larger degree of trauma energy should be suspected than in nonobese patients. Prompt initiation of antibiotic prophylaxis is of paramount importance. Irrigation and debridement should be performed in a timely fashion, leading to a clean wound with viable tissue. In most open fractures,

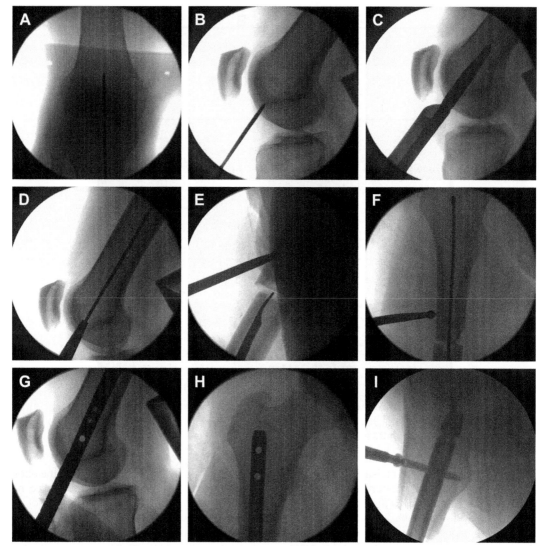

Fig. 7. Retrograde nailing technique. Anteroposterior view of the distal starting point directed from the center of the distal articular surface to the center of the femoral shaft (*A*). Lateral view showing the starting point at the anterior aspect of Blumensaat line (intercondylar fossa) directed toward the center of the femoral canal (*B*). Advancement of the guide wire and starting reamer into the proximal femur (*C*). Advancement of the ball-tipped guide wire (*D*) and reduction of the fracture using a percutaneous ball-spike pusher and an intramedullary reduction device (*E*). Advancement of the guide wire (*F*) into the proximal femur for sequential reaming. Confirmation of adequate depth of the nail at the distal (*G*) and proximal femur beyond the level of the lesser trochanter (*H*), and subsequent locking (*I*).

intramedullary nailing of the femur can proceed as a definitive procedure at initial debridement. In severe injuries and those with gross contamination, however, nailing should be performed in a delayed fashion, and may involve temporary external fixation with delayed intramedullary nailing,[62] serial debridements, and administration of local antibiotics using antibiotic beads or antibiotic cement spacers in the event of bony defects.

INTERPROSTHETIC FRACTURES

Intramedullary nailing is the preferred method of fixation of femoral shaft fractures in obese patients, given favorable biomechanical properties that allow for early weight bearing. However, in the presence of implants that preclude adequate access to the medullary canal, intramedullary nailing may not be feasible, thereby requiring plate fixation with screws and cables (**Fig. 9**).

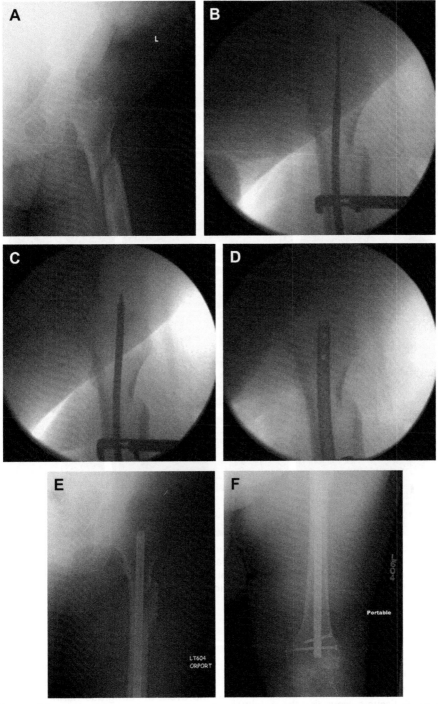

Fig. 8. A 58-year-old patient with spontaneous subtrochanteric femur fracture while standing. Due to large body habitus (BMI 57 kg/m²), an adequate proximal starting point was not deemed to be obtainable. Anteroposterior view of the proximal femur (A). After advancement of a guide wire (B) and reamer into the piriformis fossa (C), a retrograde nail was inserted (D). Proximal fracture fixation was obtained with 2 interlocking screws and interference fit of the tip in the piriformis fossa (E, F).

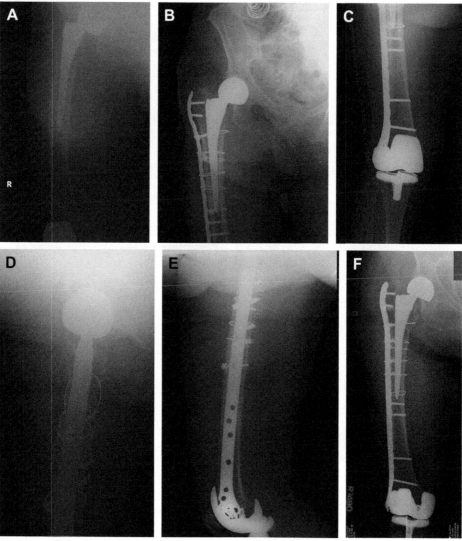

Fig. 9. A 93-year-old patient (BMI 32 kg/m²) with an interprosthetic femoral shaft fracture. Anteroposterior view of the femoral shaft fracture showing a proximal bipolar hip hemiarthroplasty and a distal total knee replacement (*A*). Postoperative anteroposterior (*B, C*) and lateral (*D, E*) views after open reduction internal fixation using a lateral locked plate, screws, and cables. Anteroposterior radiograph at 2 months after surgery (*F*).

SUMMARY

Femoral shaft fractures in obese individuals pose a significant challenge from both a diagnostic and therapeutic perspective. Because of the presence of prominent soft tissue surrounding the proximal femur, concomitant injuries to the neck and acetabulum may be difficult to identify, and frequently require CT scanning to adequately rule out these injuries. Fracture fixation should ideally be performed with intramedullary nails, given their favorable biomechanical properties compared with plates and screws. Special attention should be paid to adequate positioning and padding to reduce the risk of intraoperative complications. Retrograde nailing is the treatment of choice because it allows more expedited fixation, requiring less exposure to fluoroscopy. In the event of retrograde nailing being contraindicated, antegrade nailing should be performed through the tip of the greater trochanter to avoid extensive soft-tissue dissection required in the patient population when piriformis entry nails are used. A high degree of postoperative complication should be expected, including myocardial infarction, pneumonia, deep venous thrombosis, and wound infection.

REFERENCES

1. National Health And Nutrition Survey (NHANES). Overweight, obesity, and healthy weight among persons 20 years of age and over, according to sex, age, race, and Hispanic origin: United States, 1960–62, 1971–74, 1976–80, 1988–94, and 1999–2002. Atlanta (GA): Center for Disease Control and Prevention, National Center of Health Statistics; 2004.
2. Singh GK, Siahpush M, Kogan MD. Rising social inequalities in US childhood obesity, 2003–2007. Ann Epidemiol 2010;20(1):40–52.
3. Najjar MF, Kuczmarski RJ. Anthropometric data and prevalence of overweight for Hispanics: 1982-84. Vital Health Stat 11 1989;239:1–106.
4. Broussard BA, Sugarman JR, Bachman-Carter K, et al. Toward comprehensive obesity prevention programs in Native American communities. Obes Res 1995;3(Suppl 2):289s–97s.
5. Flegal KM, Carroll MD, Ogden CL, et al. Prevalence and trends in obesity among US adults, 1999–2000. JAMA 2002;288(14):1723–7.
6. Flegal KM, Carroll MD, Ogden CL, et al. Prevalence and trends in obesity among US adults, 1999–2008. JAMA 2010;303(3):235–41.
7. Jupiter JB, Ring D, Rosen H. The complications and difficulties of management of nonunion in the severely obese. J Orthop Trauma 1995;9(5):363–70.
8. Clinical guidelines on the identification, evaluation, and treatment of overweight and obesity in adults. Bethesda (MD): The evidence report. National Institutes of Health; 1998.
9. Maheshwari R, Mack CD, Kaufman RP, et al. Severity of injury and outcomes among obese trauma patients with fractures of the femur and tibia: a crash injury research and engineering network study. J Orthop Trauma 2009;23(9):634–9.
10. McKee MD, Waddell JP. Intramedullary nailing of femoral fractures in morbidly obese patients. J Trauma 1994;36(2):208–10.
11. Karunakar MA, Shah SN, Jerabek S. Body mass index as a predictor of complications after operative treatment of acetabular fractures. J Bone Joint Surg Am 2005;87(7):1498–502.
12. Katz DA, McHorney CA, Atkinson RL. Impact of obesity on health-related quality of life in patients with chronic illness. J Gen Intern Med 2000;15(11):789–96.
13. Leet AI, Pichard CP, Ain MC. Surgical treatment of femoral fractures in obese children: does excessive body weight increase the rate of complications? J Bone Joint Surg Am 2005;87(12):2609–13.
14. Choban PS, Heckler R, Burge JC, et al. Increased incidence of nosocomial infections in obese surgical patients. Am Surg 1995;61(11):1001–5.
15. Brown CV, Neville AL, Rhee P, et al. The impact of obesity on the outcomes of 1,153 critically injured blunt trauma patients. J Trauma 2005;59(5):1048–51 [discussion: 1051].
16. Byrnes MC, McDaniel MD, Moore MB, et al. The effect of obesity on outcomes among injured patients. J Trauma 2005;58(2):232–7.
17. Choban PS, Weireter LJ Jr, Maynes C. Obesity and increased mortality in blunt trauma. J Trauma 1991;31(9):1253–7.
18. Tucker MC, Schwappach JR, Leighton RK, et al. Results of femoral intramedullary nailing in patients who are obese versus those who are not obese: a prospective multicenter comparison study. J Orthop Trauma 2007;21(8):523–9.
19. Beck TJ, Petit MA, Wu G, et al. Does obesity really make the femur stronger? BMD, geometry, and fracture incidence in the women's health initiative-observational study. J Bone Miner Res 2009;24(8):1369–79.
20. Laasonen EM, Kivioja A. Delayed diagnosis of extremity injuries in patients with multiple injuries. J Trauma 1991;31(2):257–60.
21. Tornetta P 3rd, Kain MS, Creevy WR. Diagnosis of femoral neck fractures in patients with a femoral shaft fracture. Improvement with a standard protocol. J Bone Joint Surg Am 2007;89(1):39–43.
22. Swiontkowski MF, Hansen ST Jr, Kellam J. Ipsilateral fractures of the femoral neck and shaft. A treatment protocol. J Bone Joint Surg Am 1984;66(2):260–8.
23. Yang KH, Han DY, Park HW, et al. Fracture of the ipsilateral neck of the femur in shaft nailing. The role of CT in diagnosis. J Bone Joint Surg Br 1998;80(4):673–8.
24. Hughes SS, Voit G, Kates SL. The role of computerized tomography in the diagnosis of an occult femoral neck fracture associated with an ipsilateral femoral shaft fracture: case report. J Trauma 1991;31(2):296–8.
25. Levy BA, Zlowodzki MP, Graves M, et al. Screening for extremity arterial injury with the arterial pressure index. Am J Emerg Med 2005;23(5):689–95.
26. Lynch K, Johansen K. Can Doppler pressure measurement replace "exclusion" arteriography in the diagnosis of occult extremity arterial trauma? Ann Surg 1991;214(6):737–41.
27. Mills WJ, Barei DP, McNair P. The value of the ankle-brachial index for diagnosing arterial injury after knee dislocation: a prospective study. J Trauma 2004;56(6):1261–5.
28. Mandrella B. [The conservative treatment of femur fractures by Perkin traction. Management in adverse situations]. Unfallchirurg 2002;105(10):923–31 [in German].
29. Handolin LE, Hiltunen OJ. Perioperative difficulties in fluoroscopy of the femoral head in massive obese patient: enhanced visualization by intra-articular

contrast agent. Arch Orthop Trauma Surg 2006;126 (7):498–9.

30. Winfield RD, Delano MJ, Lottenberg L, et al. Traditional resuscitative practices fail to resolve metabolic acidosis in morbidly obese patients after severe blunt trauma. J Trauma 2010;68(2): 317–30.

31. Pape HC, Hildebrand F, Pertschy S, et al. Changes in the management of femoral shaft fractures in polytrauma patients: from early total care to damage control orthopedic surgery. J Trauma 2002;53(3): 452–61 [discussion: 461–2].

32. Bhandari M, Zlowodzki M, Tornetta P 3rd, et al. Intramedullary nailing following external fixation in femoral and tibial shaft fractures. J Orthop Trauma 2005;19(2):140–4.

33. Nowotarski PJ, Turen CH, Brumback RJ, et al. Conversion of external fixation to intramedullary nailing for fractures of the shaft of the femur in multiply injured patients. J Bone Joint Surg Am 2000;82(6): 781–8.

34. Streubel PN, Arndt S, Armitage MS, et al. Fatal knee dislocation in a morbidly obese jehovah's witness. A case report. Obes Surg 2010;20(9):1316–8.

35. Higgins TF, Horwitz DS. Damage control nailing. J Orthop Trauma 2007;21(7):477–81 [dicussion: 481–4].

36. Clatworthy MG, Clark DI, Gray DH, et al. Reamed versus unreamed femoral nails. A randomised, prospective trial. J Bone Joint Surg Br 1998;80(3): 485–9.

37. COTS. Nonunion following intramedullary nailing of the femur with and without reaming. Results of a multicenter randomized clinical trial. J Bone Joint Surg Am 2003;85(11):2093–6.

38. Winquist RA, Hansen ST Jr, Clawson DK. Closed intramedullary nailing of femoral fractures. A report of five hundred and twenty cases. J Bone Joint Surg Am 1984;66(4):529–39.

39. Wolinsky PR, McCarty E, Shyr Y, et al. Reamed intramedullary nailing of the femur: 551 cases. J Trauma 1999;46(3):392–9.

40. Tan V, Pepe MD, Glaser DL, et al. Well-leg compartment pressures during hemilithotomy position for fracture fixation. J Orthop Trauma 2000;14(3):157–61.

41. Ostrum RF. A greater trochanteric insertion site for femoral intramedullary nailing in lipomatous patients. Orthopedics 1996;19(4):337–40.

42. Tornetta P 3rd, Tiburzi D. Antegrade or retrograde reamed femoral nailing. A prospective, randomised trial. J Bone Joint Surg Br 2000;82(5):652–4.

43. Ricci WM, Bellabarba C, Evanoff B, et al. Retrograde versus antegrade nailing of femoral shaft fractures. J Orthop Trauma 2001;15(3):161–9.

44. Ostrum RF, DiCicco J, Lakatos R, et al. Retrograde intramedullary nailing of femoral diaphyseal fractures. J Orthop Trauma 1998;12(7):464–8.

45. Ostrum RF, Agarwal A, Lakatos R, et al. Prospective comparison of retrograde and antegrade femoral intramedullary nailing. J Orthop Trauma 2000;14(7): 496–501.

46. Moed BR, Watson JT, Cramer KE, et al. Unreamed retrograde intramedullary nailing of fractures of the femoral shaft. J Orthop Trauma 1998;12(5): 334–42.

47. Gregory P, DiCicco J, Karpik K, et al. Ipsilateral fractures of the femur and tibia: treatment with retrograde femoral nailing and unreamed tibial nailing. J Orthop Trauma 1996;10(5):309–16.

48. Moed BR, Watson JT. Retrograde intramedullary nailing, without reaming, of fractures of the femoral shaft in multiply injured patients. J Bone Joint Surg Am 1995;77(10):1520–7.

49. Patterson BM, Routt ML Jr, Benirschke SK, et al. Retrograde nailing of femoral shaft fractures. J Trauma 1995;38(1):38–43.

50. Sanders R, Koval KJ, DiPasquale T, et al. Retrograde reamed femoral nailing. J Orthop Trauma 1993;7(4):293–302.

51. van der Elst M, van der Werken C. Bilateral retrograde femoral nailing in an obese patient. Injury 1999;30(5):371–3.

52. Herscovici D Jr, Whiteman KW. Retrograde nailing of the femur using an intercondylar approach. Clin Orthop Relat Res 1996;332:98–104.

53. Hupel TM, Aksenov SA, Schemitsch EH. Effect of limited and standard reaming on cortical bone blood flow and early strength of union following segmental fracture. J Orthop Trauma 1998;12(6): 400–6.

54. Hupel TM, Weinberg JA, Aksenov SA, et al. Effect of unreamed, limited reamed, and standard reamed intramedullary nailing on cortical bone porosity and new bone formation. J Orthop Trauma 2001;15(1): 18–27.

55. Ricci WM, Gallagher B, Haidukewych GJ. Intramedullary nailing of femoral shaft fractures: current concepts. J Am Acad Orthop Surg 2009;17(5): 296–305.

56. Brumback RJ, Toal TR Jr, Murphy-Zane MS, et al. Immediate weight-bearing after treatment of a comminuted fracture of the femoral shaft with a statically locked intramedullary nail. J Bone Joint Surg Am 1999;81(11):1538–44.

57. Blair B, Koval KJ, Kummer F, et al. Basicervical fractures of the proximal femur. A biomechanical study of 3 internal fixation techniques. Clin Orthop Relat Res 1994;306:256–63.

58. Mallick A, Parker MJ. Basal fractures of the femoral neck: intra- or extracapsular. Injury 2004;35(10): 989–93.

59. Baitner AC, Maurer SG, Hickey DG, et al. Vertical shear fractures of the femoral neck. A biomechanical study. Clin Orthop Relat Res 1999;367:300–5.

60. Liporace F, Gaines R, Collinge C, et al. Results of internal fixation of Pauwels type-3 vertical femoral neck fractures. J Bone Joint Surg Am 2008;90(8):1654–9.

61. Deneka DA, Simonian PT, Stankewich CJ, et al. Biomechanical comparison of internal fixation techniques for the treatment of unstable basicervical femoral neck fractures. J Orthop Trauma 1997;11 (5):337–43.

62. Malik ZU, Hanif MS, Safdar A, et al. Planned external fixation to locked intramedullary nailing conversion for open fractures of shaft of femur and tibia. J Coll Physicians Surg Pak 2005;15(3):133–6.

Periarticular Tibial Fracture Treatment in the Obese Population

Matt L. Graves, MD

KEYWORDS

- Periarticular • Fracture • Obese • Tibia • Plateau
- Pilon • Plafond

Lambotte's 7 steps of fracture treatment have stood the test of time.[1] Incision, preparation of the bone ends, reduction, temporary fixation, permanent fixation, closure, and dressing are modified to suit the needs of each fracture and each patient. One specific patient characteristic, obesity, has provided complex challenges in fracture care.[2–9] This article reviews the challenges of obesity as they relate to the 7 steps of lower extremity periarticular fracture care. Specifically, helpful modifications to these 7 steps are provided for the treatment of tibial plateau fractures and tibial plafond fractures. As there is little published evidence with respect to the treatment of these injuries in the obese population, the suggestions that are provided are based on the extrapolation from published evidence of fracture care in other areas in patients with obesity, logic, and personal experience with fracture care in patients with obesity.

STEPS OF PERIARTICULAR FRACTURE CARE IN PATIENTS WITH OBESITY
Incision (Including Positioning and Approach)

A surgical incision is a means to an end in fracture care. The desired ends include visualization of the fracture, preparation of the bone ends, reduction of the fracture, and fixation of the fracture. These ends need to be accomplished in the absence of wound healing complications. Obesity complicates reaching each of these ends. Modifications

of the technique of the surgical incision are therefore useful.

Position must first be addressed as it allows access to the proposed location of the incision. Proper positioning of the patient begins at the operating room bed. Standard operating room beds may not be sufficient to allow for treatment of lower extremity periarticular fractures in the morbidly obese. Knowledge of the maximum weight allowance is necessary, which is provided in the technical specifications that come with the bed and is often listed on the bed itself. The location of the weight can be just as important as the amount of weight involved. Obesity takes different forms, and each form provides a different challenge. Truncal obesity leads to a significant shift in the patient's center of gravity when rotational adjustments are made with the bed or bumps are placed under the hip. Overcoming the exaggerated lower extremity externally rotated resting posture in the patient with obesity is challenging and often requires these rotational adjustments to be made with the bed. This adjustment necessitates diligence before preparing and draping in placement of restraints to counteract the unwanted vectors that are created by bed rotation and shifts in the center of gravity. These restraints must distribute the force over a large area to limit the stress placed on the soft tissue envelope and thereby limit skin breakdown or neuropathies created through surgical positioning. Extra large belts and belt extensions are available and logically beneficial in this population. Using more

There was no pharmaceutical or industry support or funding for this article.
Financial disclosure: The author is a paid consultant for Synthes USA.
Division of Trauma, Department of Orthopaedic Surgery and Rehabilitation, University of Mississippi Medical Center, 2500 North State Street, Jackson, MS 39216, USA
E-mail address: Mattgraves1@gmail.com

Orthop Clin N Am 42 (2011) 37–44
doi:10.1016/j.ocl.2010.08.003

than a single belt helps provide a second check-rein but should be balanced with the understanding that more pressure points are being created.

Once a bed with adequate weight allowance is chosen, modification of the bed to allow for increased width is often necessary. Thigh obesity creates an obligatory abduction at the level of the hips secondary to medial thigh abutment. This abduction increases the width of the bed required, as the limb extends distally. Once the ankles are reached, both feet may not be adequately supported. A published modification is to place an arm board distally, parallel to the long axis of the bed.[9] Although increasing bed width, this modification comes at a cost. Many arm boards are not radiolucent, creating impairments in radiographic visualization when working at or distal to the knee. This situation can be remedied in single-extremity trauma by placing the arm board under the nonoperative extremity and moving the patient slightly toward the arm board in an effort to better center the injured extremity onto the radiolucent bed. Having the arm board slightly more elevated than the bed allows for a ramp effect to decrease the risk of the patient rolling off the bed. The arm board supplementation technique creates another issue that should be evaluated before beginning the procedure. C-arm machines vary in the diameter of the geometric arm. Increasing the width of the operative field may make moving from an anteroposterior to a lateral position for radiography challenging or even impossible. Even larger-diameter c-arms are taxed by increasing the width of the operative bed (**Fig. 1**).

Once the patient is appropriately positioned and secured on a radiolucent bed of adequate dimensions and weight allowances, attention can be placed on preparing and draping. Intertriginous zones and folds must be aggressively cleansed (**Fig. 2**). Personal hygiene can often be challenging in this population, and these folds have the potential to harbor bacterial contaminants that could create postoperative wound infections. Handling an unstable extremity during the preparation may require more than one assistant for the following reasons: (1) instability is magnified by the weight of the limb, (2) preparation time may be extended to cover the additional surface area, and (3) hoisting the extra weight of the limb can lead to premature exhaustion.

After adequate preparing and draping, the surgical approach is finally possible. As previously noted, a surgical incision is a means to an end in fracture care. The desired ends include visualization of the fracture, preparation of the bone ends,

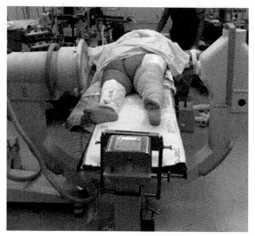

Fig. 1. Limited clearance is noted with intraoperative lateral ankle fluoroscopy using the OEC 9900 Elite Super-C (GE Healthcare, Piscataway, NJ, USA) c-arm with the arm board extension technique. This c-arm has one of the largest geometric arm diameters currently available.

reduction of the fracture, and fixation of the fracture. These ends need to be accomplished in the absence of wound healing complications. Decisions are made by balancing desires with requirements. Doing so in periarticular fracture care in patients with obesity has led to 2 different strategies. First, larger approaches have been used to allow for adequate visualization and reductions, with the acceptance of increased wound healing complications.[2–4] Second, limited incision approaches have been used in an effort to decrease wound healing complications but often at the expense of quality and construct stability. If

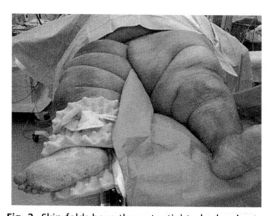

Fig. 2. Skin folds have the potential to harbor bacterial contaminants that could produce postoperative wound infections. Diligence during preparing is required. This image also reveals the exaggerated externally rotated resting posture of the lower extremity that must be overcome when making lateral and posterolateral approaches.

the first approach is chosen, every care should be taken to limit wound healing complications through atraumatic soft tissue handling, careful closure, and even possibly wound healing enhancement techniques, such as use of incisional wound vacuum-assisted closure devices.[2] If the second approach is chosen, special instrumentation, patience, and honing indirect reduction techniques should be the focus.

Preparation of the Bone Ends and Reduction

Each periarticular fracture can be divided into its component fractures: the articular fracture and the fracture that creates separation between the epiphysis and the diaphysis. The caveat to this rule is the partial articular fracture (eg, lateral tibial plateau fracture). These component fractures have different requirements and can be approached as such. It is generally accepted that the quality of a fracture reduction is inversely related to the maintenance of blood supply to the fracture fragments. It is not hard to enact an anatomic reduction if all the deforming forces (and therefore all the viability) are removed. Similarly, it is not hard to maintain soft tissue attachments if reduction is not a primary concern. To resolve this conflict, it is necessary to understand the reduction requirements of the area involved. It is generally accepted that the articular fracture component mandates an anatomic reduction in an effort to limit the risk of posttraumatic arthritis. This reduction is typically accomplished via an open (possibly extensile) approach and direct reduction techniques with visualization of the fracture reduction. In contrast, the fracture component that creates separation between the epiphysis and diaphysis has different reduction requirements. All that is typically required is a functional reduction (restoration of length, alignment, and rotation). Because of the less-stringent reduction requirement, this reduction can often be accomplished while preserving nearly all viability via a limited approach with indirect reduction techniques and radiographic confirmation of the reduction.

In the obese population, the articular reduction for tibial periarticular fractures can be challenging. Limb geometry differs greatly between the 2 populations. Open approaches to the articular surface typically have to be larger because the visual field decreases as the depth of approach increases. Adjunctive aids become even more important. The universal distractor (Synthes, WestChester, PA, USA) improves joint visualization and limits unwanted deforming forces (which are often accentuated by the increased size of the limb). A headlight is especially useful as the depth of approach increases. Once adequate visualization is present, unique reduction difficulties are encountered. Standard clamps were designed for average-sized individuals. These clamps often fit poorly in the morbidly obese population. Although the bone diameter varies little compared with the nonobese population, the soft tissue circumference varies greatly. This increase in soft tissue circumference can lead to soft tissue crushing with standard clamp designs. The excursion of a clamp and the maximum distance between the 2 arms are linked by the clamp design. Design parameters such as the clamp arm shape, the ability of the clamp to disarticulate, and the locking mechanism affect its use (**Fig. 3**). Periarticular clamps, pelvic clamps, and collinear clamps should be available when attempting tibial reductions in the obese population. When both tines of the clamp are placed through the surgical approach, periarticular designs are less beneficial and even create a disadvantage when compared with the standard clamp designs; however, when one or both tines of the clamp need to be placed through a percutaneous incision, soft tissue crushing can be prevented with these alternative clamp designs.

In the obese population, the metadiaphyseal reduction for tibial periarticular fractures is more challenging than that in nonobese patients. As previously described, the reduction requirement at this level is typically functional (restoration of length,

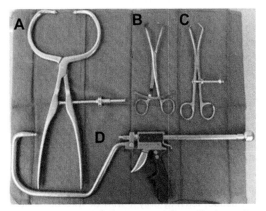

Fig. 3. Four types of clamps used for articular reductions. (*A*) Peri- articular clamp with speed-lock mechanism. (*B*) Large Weber pointed reduction clamp with ratchet locking mechanism. (*C*) Large Weber pointed reduction clamp with speed-lock mechanism. (*D*) Collinear reduction clamp. Note increased excursion and maximum possible distance between arms in (*A*) and (*D*). Clamps that allow for large excursions and large distances between arms are especially useful for morbidly obese patients when one or both tines are inserted percutaneously.

alignment, and rotation) rather than anatomic (perfect repositioning of all fragments). The less-stringent reduction requirements allow for a more limited surgical approach, which is beneficial for maintaining the fracture milieu and optimizing fragment viability. The reduction in this area is important because the cartilage stress and shear created by articular malalignment would logically be greater in the obese population. The importance of the reduction and the common choice for a limited approach mandates skill with indirect reduction techniques and fluoroscopic interpretation. Tools for regaining length, alignment, and rotation at a distance from the zone of injury include the universal distractor and the external fixator. A clear understanding of the direction of displacement allows one to create appropriate reduction vectors with these tools. Strategically placed towel bumps are useful for the correction of sagittal plane malalignment. Judiciously combining nonlocking and locking fixation can greatly ease coronal plane reduction. Knowledge of population alignment norms improves fluoroscopic interpretation. Because of the limited field of view provided with fluoroscopy, intraoperative plain films are occasionally necessary to ensure appropriate articular alignment.

Temporary and Permanent Fixation (Including Implant Selection and Mechanics)

Moving from the point of reduction to definitive stabilization can be challenging. In any patient, care must be taken to strategically place clamps and wires outside of the proposed placement of the plate. The only difference in this step as it relates to obese patients is the amount of provisional fixation required. Because the deforming loads are greater, the instruments or implants used to provisionally prevent those deforming loads also need to be stronger or more in number. In the proximal and distal tibia, this is accomplished by using more numerous wire placements. Secondary to the greater number of wires placed, alternative wire placement techniques can be helpful. Around the tibial plateau, wires can be inserted through the lateral approach and the medial soft tissue, leaving only 1 mm of wire still exiting the lateral plateau. This allows for unrestricted lateral plate placement with little concern for obstructing wires. Longer wires may be necessary with this technique to ensure that they can reach far enough to allow for extraction from the medial side. The same technique is possible around the tibial plafond, but care must be taken to keep wires away from the posteromedial neurovascular bundle and to elevate the heel and ankle from the table to prevent wire penetration into the drapes.

Another useful technique is to replace wires with minifragment screws. The flat heads of these screws allow for placement beneath plates without compromising the relationship of the plate to the underlying bone. Longer minifragment screws are available on special request.

Percutaneous insertion handles and screw hole targeting guides are commonplace. The design of these guides must be considered when treating the morbidly obese population. Standard 1-piece insertion handles and targeting guides may not allow for implant insertion secondary to the limited distance between the bone and the targeting guide and the angle of insertion required in obese patients. To clarify, the distal end of the targeting guide impinges against the extensive soft tissue envelope during insertion, preventing plate insertion. This problem can be solved by using 2-piece insertion handle/targeting guides or by increasing the length of the surgical incision. However, the incision does not need to extend to the bone. If a longer incision is chosen, the distal portion of the incision does not need to extend to the bone. An approach through the skin and adipose layer will eliminate soft tissue impingement and allow the use of standard 1-piece insertion handles.

Mechanical instabilities are magnified in the morbidly obese population. Loads are greater, so diligence is required in understanding failure modes and designing fracture fixation constructs to prevent failures. Fracture care is a race between construct failure and fracture healing. Morbid obesity complicates the race by tipping the scales toward construct failure. Construct stability depends on the bone quality, fracture pattern, reduction quality, loading technique (compression vs bridging), and implant used. As a general rule, creating a load-sharing construct is preferred. In the periarticular tibial fracture, this load sharing applies to the fracture between the epiphysis and diaphysis. As previously noted, this fracture pattern is often comminuted, such that load sharing is impossible. Therefore, more attention must be given to implant mechanics.

Partial articular tibial plateau fractures are most commonly of 2 types, the lateral split depression type and the medial fracture dislocation type. In the lateral split depression type, instability may be divided into 2 types: (1) axial subsidence and (2) valgus malalignment. Both of these are most logically treated with a lateral nonlocking plate construct. Three points of the construct must be addressed. First, a subchondral raft of screws or Kirschner wires should be placed either in the osteochondral fragments or immediately caudal to them. Second, a nonlocking screw should be placed immediately below the split to allow the plate to appropriately serve as a buttress. Third, the metaphyseal impaction void should be filled with a bone-grafting substitute (**Fig. 4**). Recently, calcium phosphate cement has been touted in both clinical and biomechanical studies to have better resistance to axial subsidence.[10,11] Care must be taken when using this substitute to ensure that it does not escape into the articular surface through articular incongruities. The medial fracture dislocation type is more complicated because it commonly occurs in conjunction with knee ligament abnormalities. Medial implants are preferred in this fracture type (**Fig. 5**). Lateral locked implants are incapable of reducing the deformity and stabilize the deformity only through the limited screw capture into the medial fragment.

Complete articular tibial plateau fractures are of many types, but varus displacement is of the most concern. Postoperative varus displacement is typically resisted in 2 ways: (1) lateral locked implants and (2) lateral and posteromedial plating via dual approaches. This fracture is a complex topic and is beyond the scope of this article. To simplify and summarize, dual plating has been shown in mechanical studies to provide more resistance to varus displacement.[12] As the loads increase in the morbidly obese population, this added resistance may become clinically relevant, which is unproven and is only a logical conjecture. The consequence of choosing dual plating is an additional surgical exposure through an obese envelope. The risk of incisional complications around the knee in the morbidly obese population is unknown.

Tibial plafond failure modes vary. As in tibial plateau fractures, the initial injury radiographs clearly depict the deforming forces. With the advances in implant design for fractures around the ankle, implant placement can be tailored to help resist failure. Although there is little biomechanical evidence to support this line of thought, it is simple to extrapolate from what is available. Valgus and anterior translational deforming forces are logically treated with an anterolateral implant (**Fig. 6**), which places the strength of the fixation in the correct place to resist the deforming forces.

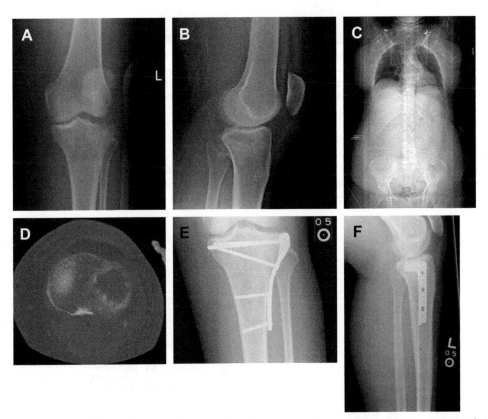

Fig. 4. Addressing instability in lateral split depression tibial plateau fractures. (*A, B*) Anteroposterior (AP) and lateral radiographs of the injury. (*C*) Computed tomographic (CT) scout image noting truncal obesity. (*D*) CT axial view denoting impaction defect. (*E, F*) AP and lateral radiographs at 2-month follow-up. Note the subchondral raft of screws, the screw placed at the apex of the split, and the bone graft substitute placed in the defect created by the metaphyseal impaction.

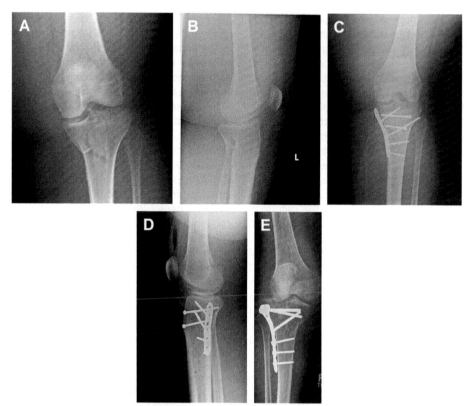

Fig. 5. Addressing instability in a medial plateau fracture dislocation. (*A, B*) Anteroposterior (AP) and lateral radiographs of the injury. Note the femur remains in a relationship with the medial plateau, but the remainder of the leg is displaced. (*C, D*) Postoperative AP and lateral radiographs denoting restoration of alignment. (*E*) A different case revealing an unsuccessful attempt to treat a medial fracture dislocation with a lateral locked implant.

Bicortical screws placed in the anterolateral shaft help anchor the implant to the strongest part of the bone, limiting the ability of the talus to escape in the anterolateral direction. Similarly, varus and medial translational deforming forces are logically treated with a medial implant (**Fig. 7**). Posterior translational deforming forces are more complicated to address. A posterior buttress implant requires a compromise in visualization of the articular surface. For all tibial plafond injury patterns,

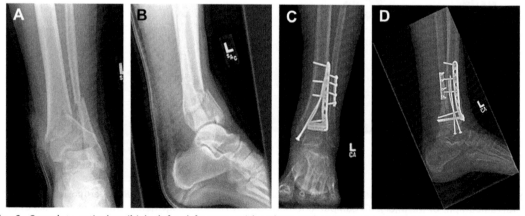

Fig. 6. Complete articular tibial plafond fracture with valgus and anterior translational displacement treated with an anterolateral implant. (*A, B*) Anteroposterior (AP) and lateral radiographs of the injury. (*C, D*) Follow-up AP and lateral imaging.

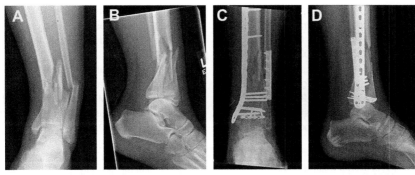

Fig. 7. Complete articular tibial plafond fracture with varus and medial translational displacement treated with a medial implant. (*A, B*) Anteroposterior (AP) and lateral radiographs of the injury. (*C, D*) Follow-up AP and lateral imaging.

the optimal mechanical choice must be tempered by an understanding of the soft tissue injury and the needed visualization to enact an articular reduction.

Closure and Dressing (Including Postoperative Protocol)

Meticulous closure is the standard of care in periarticular trauma. Because of the higher wound healing complication rate noted in other areas of the body in obese patients, greater attention to detail would be paid to treatment in this area as well. The only series available comparing obese with nonobese patients with respect to open plating of tibial plafond fractures noted a similar incidence in wound healing complications, with a trend toward more problems in the obese population.[8]

The poorly vascularized subcutaneous fat layer is likely the problem, but attention should be focused on all aspects of closure. Creating a deep-layer seal is advantageous in case superficial healing complications arise. Taking tension off the damaged skin envelope can be accomplished via special suture techniques (eg, Allgower modification of the Donati technique).[13] Placement of incisional vacuum-assisted closure devices has been shown to be advantageous in fracture surgery in the obese pelvic and acetabular region.[2] This technique would be beneficial in periarticular lower extremity fracture care in the obese population, although not yet proven.

Prophylactic antibiotic use has changed slightly in the author's treatment of obese patients. Specifically, the dosing of antibiotics depends on the larger soft tissue envelope available for distribution.[14] In the obese population, loading dose cefazolin is given in 2-g doses rather than in 1-g doses. This increased dosing has been supported in the abdominal surgical literature.[14] There is no literature to support the use of antibiotics for longer than 24 hours postoperatively in routine fracture care.[15,16] Although

increased dosing could potentially decrease the incidence of postoperative wound infections resulting from secondary contamination, it could also increase the incidence of resistant bacteria. The author does not believe that the potential benefit would outweigh the potential risk and continues to use the standard duration of perioperative antibiotics.

The postoperative rehabilitation protocol has varied little with respect to obesity. As loads are greater and postoperative mobilization is generally more complicated, strict attention must be paid to weight-bearing precautions. In-hospital time is often longer in this group because of mobilization issues. Weight bearing is delayed until there are radiographic signs of healing. For periarticular lower extremity fracture care, this time varies greatly. The author's standard has nonetheless been the same for the obese and nonobese populations, beginning weight bearing at approximately 10 to 12 weeks and advancing on a progressive basis.

SUMMARY

Periarticular fracture care in the morbidly obese population is challenging. Modifications of Lambotte's 7 steps of fracture treatment have been helpful in solving some of the challenges encountered. Despite all these helpful modifications, maintaining a positive attitude is the greatest challenge. Entering into a surgical encounter with a morbidly obese patient requires optimism and focus, which can be hard to muster with the understanding that the same surgical procedure, if performed on a nonobese patient, would likely require less time, cause less frustration, and have a lower incidence of wound healing complications.

REFERENCES

1. Seligson D. Lambotte's "seven steps" for osteosynthesis. Techniques in Orthopaedics 1986;1:10–2.

2. Reddix RN Jr, Tyler HK, Kulp B, et al. Incisional vacuum-assisted wound closure in morbidly obese patients undergoing acetabular fracture surgery. Am J Orthop (Belle Mead NJ) 2009;38:446–9.

3. Porter SE, Russell GV, Dews RC, et al. Complications of acetabular fracture surgery in morbidly obese patients. J Orthop Trauma 2008;22:589–94.

4. Karunakar MA, Shah SN, Jerabek S. Body mass index as a predictor of complications after operative treatment of acetabular fractures. J Bone Joint Surg Am 2005;87:1498–502.

5. Bostman OM. Body-weight related to loss of reduction of fractures of the distal tibia and ankle. J Bone Joint Surg Br 1995;77:101–3.

6. Sems SA, Johnson M, Cole PA, et al. Elevated body mass index increases early complications of surgical treatment of pelvic ring injuries. J Orthop Trauma 2010;24:309–14.

7. Porter SE, Graves ML, Qin Z, et al. Operative experience of pelvic fractures in the obese. Obes Surg 2008;18:702–8.

8. Graves ML, Porter SE, Fagan BC, et al. Is obesity protective against wound healing complications in pilon surgery? Soft tissue envelope and pilon fractures in the obese. Orthopedics 2010;33:625–7.

9. DeOrio JK. Extending the width of an operating table using armboards. Orthopedics 2005;28:367.

10. Russell TA, Leighton RK. Comparison of autogenous bone graft and endothermic calcium phosphate cement for defect augmentation in tibial plateau fractures. A multicenter, prospective, randomized study. J Bone Joint Surg Am 2008; 90:2057–61.

11. Trenholm A, Landry S, McLaughlin K, et al. Comparative fixation of tibial plateau fractures using alpha-BSM, a calcium phosphate cement, versus cancellous bone graft. J Orthop Trauma 2005;19:698–702.

12. Higgins TF, Klatt J, Bachus KN. Biomechanical analysis of bicondylar tibial plateau fixation: how does lateral locking plate fixation compare to dual plate fixation? J Orthop Trauma 2007;21: 301–6.

13. Sagi HC, Papp S, Dipasquale T. The effect of suture pattern and tension on cutaneous blood flow as assessed by laser Doppler flowmetry in a pig model. J Orthop Trauma 2008;22:171–5.

14. Forse RA, Karam B, MacLean LD, et al. Antibiotic prophylaxis for surgery in morbidly obese patients. Surgery 1989;106:750–6 [discussion: 756–7].

15. Boxma H, Broekhuizen T, Patka P, et al. Randomised controlled trial of single-dose antibiotic prophylaxis in surgical treatment of closed fractures: the Dutch trauma trial. Lancet 1996;347: 1133–7.

16. Holtom PD. Antibiotic prophylaxis: current recommendations. J Am Acad Orthop Surg 2006;14: S98–100.

Ankle Injuries and Fractures in the Obese Patient

Sonia Chaudhry, MD[a], Kenneth A. Egol, MD[b],*

KEYWORDS

- Ankle • Obese • Fracture • Overweight

Ankle fractures are a common orthopedic injury, occurring at an annual incidence of 187 fractures per 100,000 people.[1] Certain ankle injuries have been associated with patient demographics such as obesity and smoking.[2] Unlike fractures of the distal radius, hip, and spine, osteoporosis does not seem to be a major risk factor for ankle fractures.[2,3] A study of more than 3500 patients with ankle fracture revealed their average body mass index (BMI), calculated as the weight in kilograms divided by height in meters squared, to be higher than the general population across all age and gender categories.[4] Naturally, these injuries affect the lower extremity mobility significantly, which itself is a risk factor for obesity. Although overweight adults with disabilities are generally as likely to attempt weight loss as those without disabilities, overweight adults having difficulty walking or using a mobility aid are the exception.[5] In part, this stems from physicians not counseling this population on the importance of physical exercise. Physicians may focus more on diet than exercise in light of limited mobility; however, recent studies suggest that reduced energy expenditure is more causative than increased food intake in the development of obesity.[6]

The implications to one's health of being overweight are numerous. More than 80% of type 2 diabetes can be attributed to obesity, which may also account for many diabetes-related deaths.[7] The association between diabetes and complications of ankle injuries has been well documented.[8–13] In addition, obesity has been associated with an increased risk of deep vein thrombosis (DVT) and pulmonary embolus (PE),[7] which are concerns with any lower extremity injury. Finally, obesity syndrome predisposes patients to osteoarthritis by altering cartilage and bone metabolism independent of weight bearing, as evidenced by the involvement of non-weight-bearing joints. The tibiotalar joint is subject to joint reaction forces of 4.5 times the body weight during walking and 10 times the body weight with running.[14] Posttraumatic arthritis in the setting of a biologic predilection for osteoarthritis can be devastating to mobility. Although there may be some protective effect of obesity on bones, with recent evidence showing that leptin resistance in obese individuals may have a favorable effect on bone mass,[15] ankle injuries in the setting of obesity are fraught with complications.

EPIDEMIOLOGY

Data on ankle injuries in the obese population require well-defined parameters of obesity. Technically, overweight refers solely to excess body weight, whereas obesity is excess fat.[16] The 2 commonly used definitions are ideal body weight, based on one's height and gender, and BMI, which correlates with body fat and relatively unaffected by height. A study of 314 ankle fractures over a 3-year period revealed 39% of cases to have resulted from slips and falls in obese individuals,

The authors have nothing to disclose.
[a] Department of Orthopaedic Surgery, NYU Hospital for Joint Diseases, 301 East 17th Street, Room 1402, New York, NY 10003, USA
[b] Department of Orthopaedic Surgery, NYU Hospital for Joint Diseases, 301 East 17th Street, Room 1402, New York, NY 10003, USA
* Corresponding author.
E-mail address: Kenneth.egol@nyumc.org

Orthop Clin N Am 42 (2011) 45–53
doi:10.1016/j.ocl.2010.07.003

defined as greater than 120% ideal body weight,[1] compared with a general prevalence of obesity less than 20% at the time of study.[17] The study also demonstrated almost double the prevalence of diabetes in the cohort with ankle injuries than would be expected in the general population. The latest data compiled in 2008 detailed an obesity rate (BMI>30) of 33.8% in the United States among those aged 18 years and older, with 68% being overweight (BMI>25).[18] Another retrospective review of 279 ankle fractures reported a similar increased incidence of concomitant obesity, with 35.5% incidence in patients with BMI greater than 30.[19]

Fracture pattern also seems to be affected by obesity. Although sustaining an open versus closed injury for distal tibial fractures does not seem to be a consequence of body mass,[20] obese individuals were more likely to sustain Orthopaedic Trauma Association[21] type B and C fractures, and less likely to have type A fractures than nonobese patients, at rates of 1% and 11%, respectively.[19] Furthermore, the mean BMI of patients with displaced fractures is significantly higher than those with nondisplaced fractures, with one study demonstrating 83% of displaced fractures in overweight patients. Almost one-third of patients with displacement had a BMI more than 30, whereas only 1 of 24 significantly obese patients had a nondisplaced fracture.[22]

PERIOPERATIVE CONSIDERATIONS

Given the high prevalence of obesity in patients with type 2 diabetes,[7] one must pay particular attention to the risks and benefits of surgery in this specific population. There has been much data to contradict the misconception that increased surgical risks in the diabetic population should influence one toward or against operative management of ankle injuries.[7] A study of 42 closed ankle fractures in diabetic patients with matched controls demonstrated that surgery was not associated with an increased risk of infection and nonsurgical treatment did not increase the risk of malunion, nonunion, or Charcot neuroarthropathy.[10] Another source suggests that closed treatment of unstable ankle fractures is less likely to be successful in obese patients due to sporadic accidental moments of early full weight bearing.[23] In light of conflicting evidence and advances in perioperative patient care, management decisions should be based on standard parameters such as fracture pattern and ability to undergo surgery.

From the surgical booking to the postoperative splinting, once a decision is made between the surgeon and patient to undergo operative management, there are considerations specific to the obese population. Often a preoperative medical assessment or anesthesia evaluation is undertaken, in which a patient is deemed a reasonable candidate for surgery and medically optimized. An important part of optimization for obese patients with concomitant diabetes is appropriate glucose management. Tight blood glucose control has traditionally been advocated,[24] although recent evidence suggests that occasional hypoglycemia associated with lower level of hemoglobin A_{1c} may actually increase cardiovascular risks.[25] In addition, with obese individuals having a higher incidence of coronary artery disease, they may be on an anticoagulant such as aspirin. The surgeon should assess for such medication use when evaluating the patient and planning surgery. It is the authors' general practice to hold aspirin intake for 1 week before the date of surgery and restart it on the first postoperative day, although this practice is adjusted in extenuating circumstances such as high cardiac risk or intraoperative bleeding concerning for hematoma formation. If there is a medical contraindication to a period without anticoagulation preoperatively or if bleeding risks or renal function preclude the use of postoperative chemoprophylaxis, a retrievable inferior vena cava filter can be placed for interim protection from PE. One study examined the use of retrievable filters in orthopedic patients, including patients with ankle fractures, and demonstrated no complications of insertion and successful retrieval in 64% of patients.[26] Reasons for leaving filters in place include thrombosis around the filter and filter incorporation into the vessel wall, each occurring at a rate of 8%. Another consideration is comorbidities such as sleep apnea, which may require specialized equipment such as positive airway pressure machines, precluding the use of ambulatory surgery facilities if unequipped or possibly mandating an overnight stay in the hospital for monitoring.

Specialized operating room equipment and additional staff may need to be requested ahead of time. Bookings may need to include extended block time for fracture cases involving morbidly obese patients, because cases can take double the standard operative time, much of which may be spent in positioning.[27] Standard operating room tables support a maximum of 205 kg, although extrawide tables capable of holding up to 455 kg are available.[28] Position is an important consideration, primarily because the obese patient poorly tolerates poses that restrict chest or abdominal motion because they can compromise ventilation. This positioning may affect surgical approach because a surgeon preferring a posterior approach in prone position may want to consider a lateral approach in the better-tolerated lateral decubitus position, with the bulk of the panniculus adiposus displaced off the abdomen. Meticulous attention should be given to padding pressure points during positioning because obese patients are more prone to neural injuries.[23] Peroneal compartment syndrome can result from the lateral decubitus position in the dependent leg.[23] If a tourniquet is used, there are several pearls to application on the large thigh to prevent slipping or a venous tourniquet. An assistant can hold or pull back the soft tissue distally as one applies a tourniquet that ideally overlaps only a couple inches at the edges. When the soft tissue is released, it helps hold the tourniquet in place. Most commonly the authors use a supine position with the normal leg padded and the affected limb elevated on a soft foam pad (**Fig. 1**).

Choice of anesthetic is also influenced by body mass. Although regional anesthesia is associated with higher rates of block failure and complications, stemming from difficulty locating landmarks and using longer needles, overall failure rates remain low. If general anesthesia is used, rapid induction is paramount in this population with an inherently high risk of aspiration. Similar to the method of anesthesia, no definitive recommendations exist for antibiotic prophylaxis in patients undergoing foot and ankle surgery. The authors think that appropriate preoperative antibiotics should be given, although standard dosing should be adjusted. The current recommendations are to increase preoperative dosing to 2 g of cefazolin for patients weighing more than 80 kg, administer antibiotics 1 hour before incision (2 hours for vancomycin), complete the infusion before tourniquet inflation, and readminister cefazolin every 2 to 5 hours (6–12 hours for vancomycin).[29] Paiement

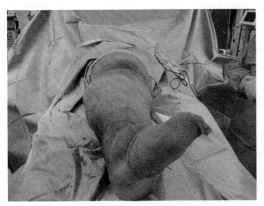

Fig. 1. Supine positioning of an obese patient using a foam pad to elevate the injured leg for both padding and intraoperative fluoroscopy access.

and colleagues[30] showed no difference in infection rates with or without the use of preoperative antibiotics in 122 patients undergoing open reduction internal fixation of closed ankle fractures in a double-blind, randomized, prospective study; however, the study may have been underpowered. A meta-analysis of more than 8000 patients demonstrated single-dose antibiotic prophylaxis to significantly lower the surgical site infections in patients undergoing surgery for several types of closed fractures, with no superior results from multiple doses.[31] For standard closed ankle fractures, the authors' practice is to use preoperative antibiotics alone for ambulatory surgery patients and to continue parenteral antibiotics for less than 24 hours for patients requiring overnight hospital stay. Lastly, skin preparation should be meticulous because obese patients are more prone to surgical site infections.

SURGICAL CONSIDERATIONS

One of the first operative considerations is the surgical approach. Although usually dependent on fracture pattern and operator preference, obese patients mandate additional consideration. Areas of active dermatitis or maceration from splinting should be avoided if possible, because wound healing may be compromised. Undermining of subcutaneous tissue should be avoided; instead, full thickness skin flaps can be used.[32] Longer incisions are often required to gain adequate exposure,[33] and multiple incisions may be called for if additional fixation is necessary to prevent loss of reduction. A Finnish study demonstrated the relative risk of loss of reduction (both for closed and open reductions) requiring surgical correction is greater than 3 for patients with a BMI greater than 1 SD above average. In this study, 1 SD above average is still less than a BMI of 30,[34] suggesting that this value may underestimate the risk in an American population. Supplemental fixation in the form of stronger plates, additional plates, locking screws, or even combining internal and external fixation can counteract this tendency toward failure. Hardware may need to cross uninvolved joints to provide a more-stable construct,[32] however, this is undesirable given the potential of joint stiffness.

Although propensity for failed reduction may stem in part from obese patients sustaining relatively more severe malleolar fractures, additional factors may be causative. Obese patients are subject to increased stress across the fracture site by noncompliance with weight-bearing status caused by impaired control of posture and physical demands of ambulating on crutches. Awareness of the increased risk of failure may help avoid failure by preemptive supplemental fixation as well as by longer periods of non-weight bearing,[12] because overweight patients may be unable to comply with partial weight bearing. Rehabilitation may be inhibited in the short term; however, this is usually outweighed by the potential prevention of malunion and reoperation.[34] Amongst obese patients, specific populations that are at increased risk for hardware failure and subsequent loss of reduction include those with diabetic neuropathy. Fracture healing time in patients with known peripheral neuropathy is 2 to 3 times longer than expected, and with 10% of diabetic patients having neuropathy at the time of diagnosis, with an additional 40% developing it within a decade, peripheral neuropathy is an important condition to screen for. Some suggest supplemental fixation for all diabetic patients.[35] Recent evidence suggests that the use of platelet rich plasma may normalize healing time in diabetic subjects[36]; however, definitive data are currently lacking.

Another method of addressing inability to comply with non-weight bearing while avoiding troublesome casting is to use external fixation.[37] One case report describes a 32-year-old obese man with an inferior tibiofibular syndesmotic injury initially fixed with tricortical 4.5-mm small fragment screws. Unable to comply with non-weightbearing due to body habitus, patient had screw backout and syndesmotic widening at 6 weeks. Two-ring Ilizarov fixators were used to reduce the syndesmosis with gradual tensioning of 2 olive wires with washers while in maximal dorsiflexion. Patient was allowed to weight bear as tolerated, and at 12 weeks, all hardware was removed. A 3-year follow-up demonstrated the patient to have maintained a reduced mortise.

Just as important as strong fixation is meticulous closure. Increased occurrence of surgical site infections is well known to be associated with obesity, especially with concomitant diabetes, and is extensively documented in both the orthopedic and general surgery literature. Postoperative hematoma may contribute to this phenomenon, because increased dead space and extensive subcutaneous tissue make this population more susceptible.[38] Scrupulous hemostasis with electrocautery, while limiting excessive devascularization of already poorly perfused tissue, as well as emphasis on elevation postoperatively may counteract this occurrence. Neither subcutaneous drains nor suturing into fat layers has shown any benefit in reducing infection rates, and it is not the authors' practice to use either because it may risk tracking bacteria into the wound or fat necrosis, respectively.

Data comparing suturing techniques for ankle injuries are limited; however, information extracted from other injuries and conditions may be applicable to ankle injuries. A study of patients with calcaneus fractures who underwent open reduction internal fixation revealed the following risk factors for wound complication: high BMI, extended time between injury and surgery, smoking, and a single-layered wound closure.[39] Although high BMI cannot be addressed acutely, physicians can expedite operative fixation when indicated, counsel patients to quit smoking, and use a 2-layered closure. Because infection is a concern with braided sutures, a monofilament should be considered for subcutaneous layer closure. The general surgery literature has shown reduced infection rates using a continuous subcutaneous monofilament closure when compared with interrupted closure in abdominal surgery in morbidly obese patients,[40] and although there is lack of orthopedic data and personal experience with this technique during ankle surgery, multiple surgeons at the authors' institution use continuous fascial and subcuticular closure techniques during hip and knee surgery with the goal of reducing infection. In addition, because wound tension is known to increase tissue pressure and reduce musculofascial microperfusion and oxygen availability for optimal healing and host defense,[41] tension-free closure is especially paramount in the obese population with swelling and edematous excess subcutaneous tissue. Higher ratios of suture length to wound length are associated with improved wound healing and should be used in the form of mattress sutures if necessary. One suture advocated is the Allgower modification of the Donati vertical mattress suture. This suture has been shown to minimize trauma to the skin of the lower leg during fracture surgery because it grasps the dermis on only one side.[42]

The authors' practice is to apply a tourniquet but defer from inflating it unless necessary. This step allows for visualization of bleeding vessels requiring electrocautery as they are encountered, minimizing postoperative hematoma formation. Furthermore, avoiding tourniquet use in these patients minimizes ischemia reperfusion injury to the tissues. Fascia is closed with an absorbable suture, subcutaneous sutures are avoided, and skin is closed in a single layer of nylon mattress sutures.

IMMOBILIZATION

With or without surgery, the obese patient is subject to difficulty with immobilization during the healing phase. Although studies focusing on immobilization in obese patients are lacking, a small study of closed ankle fractures in diabetic patients showed infection with cast treatment to occur in 4 of 6 diabetic patients versus 0 of 5 nondiabetic patients.[9] Although an infection rate of 67% should not be expected, both diabetic and obese patients are subject to fluctuating edema that imparts shear pressure from the cast leading to skin complications, and unnoticed skin breaches are likely to become infected. A warm and moist environment inside the cast is well suited for bacteria and fungus, and obese patients with fragile and poorly vascularized skin are more likely to develop abrasions and breakdown.

A practice of initial splint immobilization for the acute injury or immediate postoperative period allows some room for swelling and easier inspection of the skin at the follow-up visit (**Fig. 2**). In patients managed non operatively, the splint can then be changed to a cast, with exquisite detail paid to good casting techniques, such as well-padded edges and bony prominences along with supracalcaneal molding to limit shear forces from motion. In postoperative patients, the treated limb may be switched directly into a removable boot to allow for better hygiene; however, in a population with inherent difficulty with non-weight-bearing compliance, this switch can encourage loading of the extremity. In addition, although prefabricated boots are custom fit, the conical shape of larger ankles may not be congruent in the orthosis, and custom-molded splints may be preferable. Similar to the nonobese patient, the obese patient should be educated on the importance of adhering to an extended course of restricted weight bearing, although range of motion exercises can commence early.

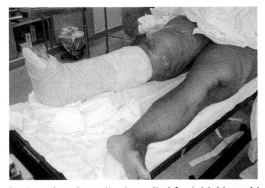

Fig. 2. A short leg splint is applied for initial immobilization and allows for inspection of skin for swelling. Note the positioning in neutral dorsiflexion and molding, which can be difficult in obese patients.

POSTOPERATIVE CONSIDERATIONS

Given the increased incidence of complications and adverse events associated with ankle surgery in the obese population, surgeons' typical postoperative protocols should be accordingly amended. Obesity is an independent risk factor for DVT and PE; therefore, anticoagulation, early ambulation, and hydration are paramount. Although there is no definitive recommendation for prophylaxis in isolated extremity trauma in general, each patient should be risk stratified and choice of prophylaxis made accordingly. Cases in which mechanoprophylaxis with sequential compression devices and/or compression stockings would otherwise be considered adequate may be indicated to have additional chemoprophylaxis. A recent review suggests supplementing with pharmacoprophylaxis for patients older than 60 years or obese patients older than 40 years with long leg casting.[23]

Early ambulation is assisted by adequate pain control. Obese patients given epidural morphine as opposed to intramuscular morphine may tolerate more vigorous physiotherapy postoperatively, leading to fewer pulmonary complications from bed rest.[38] Another option for inpatients is patient controlled analgesia. Morphine dosing should be based on ideal body weight and not on actual weight or surface area, because overmedicating patients can result in both limited mobility and decreased oxygen saturation in a population already prone to obesity hypoventilation syndrome from the inability to fully depress the diaphragm secondary to abdominal adipose tissue. In fact, much of the increased mortality associated with blunt trauma in the severely overweight patients is secondary to pulmonary issues,[43] and nursing orders such as head-of-bed elevation and chest physical therapy may benefit this population after ankle injuries. Nurses along with other health professionals can significantly contribute to the specialized care of the morbidly obese patient.

Several assistants may be needed for postoperative mobilization of and therapy for obese patients. Other potential limiting factors may include gowns not adequately covering their body habitus or poor grooming, leading a patient to want to maintain dignity with privacy in bed. Increased bed rest in this population brings up the issue of pressure-related injuries. The morbidly obese patients with lower extremity injuries are unable to reposition themselves and can have accelerated ulcer development from prolonged recumbency on poorly vascularized adipose tissue. Frequent turning and bariatric beds with low air-loss surface can prevent these complications. Patients in the intensive care unit who cannot be turned should instead have extremities frequently repositioned. In addition, while the operated leg should be elevated, the contralateral extremity should have the heels floated with a roll positioned proximally, because the heel is the second most common site of pressure ulcers.[38]

OUTCOMES

Even milder ankle injuries tend to have prolonged recovery periods in obese patients. A study of ankle sprains in patients aged 8 to 18 years demonstrated those with BMI above the 85th percentile to be more likely to have persistent symptoms at 6 months postinjury.[44] Obese patients with ankle fractures are subject to a similar course of prolonged healing, and an extended period of non-weight bearing in this population is cumbersome, given their difficulty with crutch use. Although casting is especially poorly tolerated in these cases, placement of the limb into removable braces, while allowing for range of motion, often encourages noncompliance with weight-bearing restrictions. Premature weight bearing is most likely the greatest contributing factor to the higher rates of loss of reduction. Infection rates in many studies are similarly elevated, although much of the literature focuses on infection in the diabetic patient, and one study limited to obese patients demonstrated no difference in infection rate, time to union, or complications as compared with nonobese patients.[19]

Regarding open injuries, no large studies exist specific to the obese population. A study of pilon fractures has displayed an equivalent rate of open injuries between diabetic and nondiabetic patients,[20] with diabetic patients experiencing a similar rate of wound complications but higher rates of deep infection and delayed or no union. A series specific to open ankle fractures in a cohort of 14 diabetic patients demonstrated 9 (64%) wound-healing complications, 6 (42%) eventual below-knee amputations, 5 (36%) deep infections, and only 3 (21%) bony unions without complications. These patients required an average of 5 surgeries (range, 2–10) over their course of treatment.[11] Clearly, an open ankle injury in this population with compromised healing potential is often a devastating injury with a prolonged treatment course.

Overall, obese patients require much additional care in terms of prolonged hospital stay, additional staff, increased length of therapy, and specialized assistive devices and home equipment. They often require prolonged follow-up, and development of complications begins the process anew. According to the health maintenance organization data, when compared with those with a BMI of 20 to 24.9, the mean annual total costs of patients with a BMI between 30 and 34.9 is 25% higher and increased to 44% for those with a BMI greater than 35.[9] National health care is focusing on cutting costs, and nothing seems as ubiquitous of an answer as reducing obesity in America. People with a normal BMI at present have a 25% to 30% chance of becoming obese and more than a 50% chance of becoming overweight within 30 years; even the 4-year rate of becoming overweight is up to 30% for men.[6]

AN ILLUSTRATIVE CASE

A 41-year-old obese man, with a BMI of 63 and a weight of almost 200 kg presented 4 days after fixation of a pronation external rotation injury to the left ankle with syndesmotic injury that was sustained from a mechanical fall. The patient admitted to walking on the limb. Radiographs on presentation revealed failed syndesmotic fixation, a broken screw, widening of the syndesmosis, and a minimally displaced proximal fibula fracture. The patient was indicated for revision reduction and fixation (**Fig. 3**). After medical clearance for a history of hypertension and obstructive sleep apnea, patient was taken for revision fixation. Patient was placed supine and tourniquet was applied. Prior lateral incision was opened and extended proximally, and both hardware and scar tissue were removed. Cultures were taken for completeness, although infection was neither suspected nor shown. Reduction was achieved with a King Tong clamp in neutral ankle flexion and confirmed with fluoroscopy. Decision was made to use a 5-hole plate to act as a large washer along the distal fibula, and a nonlocking 50-mm cortical screw was used with tricortical purchase. This step was followed by the insertion of two 60-mm locking screws through the plate and a final 3.5-mm nonlocking screw parallel to the joint distally. Intraoperative fluoroscopy again confirmed satisfactory reduction and hardware placement, and the leg was placed into a long leg cast with the knee in 30° flexion to prevent accidental weight bearing.

Despite the involvement of multiple assistants and meticulous attention to casting technique, the patient complained of significant cast irritation and admitted to resting the cast on the ground and occasionally bearing weight on it. After 3 weeks of operation, the patient demanded a short leg cast, into which the leg was placed against medical advice because his long leg cast had broken

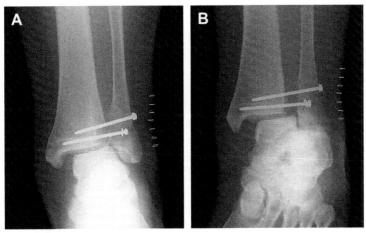

Fig. 3. A 45-year-old man with a BMI of 35 presents 2 weeks after ankle fracture repair. (*A*) Anteroposterior and (*B*) mortise views demonstrating failed fixation with a widened syndesmosis and broken hardware.

down at the footplate. The patient had multiple areas of skin maceration from ambulating on wet surfaces as well as open skin lesions from cast irritation to overhanging pannus. He limited weight bearing to the best of his ability but did not manage the use of crutches to assist him. Despite the inability to comply with weight-bearing restrictions, the patient remained reduced with intact hardware throughout his recovery period. After 8 weeks of operation, the patient presented again with cast irritation as he had showered in his short leg cast, and the leg was then placed into a walking boot. A week later, the patient had an episode of increased foot swelling and was found to have an occluding thrombus in the superficial femoral vein of the operated leg, extending to the popliteal vein, despite having been on daily aspirin. The patient was admitted for anticoagulation with warfarin (Coumadin) bridged with fondaparinux. His surgical incision was well healed. At almost 3 months postoperation, the patient was weight bearing without loss of reduction or hardware failure and was relatively pain free (**Fig. 4**).

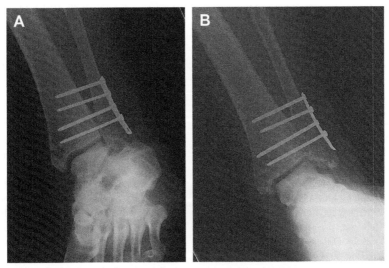

Fig. 4. Postoperative radiographs. (*A*) Mortise and (*B*) anteroposterior of the same patient from **Fig. 3** after revision surgery, demonstrating a reduced ankle mortise with intact syndesmotic screws held by plate acting as a washer.

SUMMARY

Obese patients are more prone to severe ankle injuries, and although they have increased complications across the board, there are specific techniques that can be used to assure the best possible outcome. Nonoperative management of these patients may seem like an attractive option in light of the morbidity associated with surgery, but with higher rates of loss of reduction, difficulty in tolerating casting, and inability to comply with weight-bearing restrictions, operative treatment still plays a major role. Preoperative planning should include consideration of operative table, ideal positioning, choice of anesthesia, preoperative antibiotic prophylaxis, and incisional planning. Operative considerations include supplemental fixation, meticulous closure, and immobilization. Postoperatively, patients should be adequately anticoagulated and mobilized early, with the assistance of pain control agents and skilled nurses and therapists, to prevent pulmonary complications. Increased complexity associated with the care of the morbidly obese patients with ankle injuries may seem daunting; however, the increased complication rates in these patients makes them well suited for the future study of technical factors to improve outcome. These principles can then be used to facilitate improved quality of life in obese and nonobese patients alike.

REFERENCES

1. Daly PJ, Fitzgerald RH Jr, Melton LJ, et al. Epidemiology of ankle fractures in Rochester, Minnesota. Acta Orthop Scand 1987;58(5):539–44.
2. Valtola A, Honkanen R, Kröger H, et al. Lifestyle and other factors predict ankle fractures in perimenopausal women: a population-based prospective cohort study. Bone 2002;30(1):238–42.
3. Seeley DG, Kelsey J, Jergas M, et al. Predictors of ankle and foot fractures in older women. The study of osteoporotic fractures research group. J Bone Miner Res 1996;11(9):1347–55.
4. Bostman OM. Body mass index of patients with elbow and ankle fractures requiring surgical treatment. J Trauma 1994;37(1):62–5.
5. Weil E, Wachterman M, McCarthy EP, et al. Obesity among adults with disabling conditions. JAMA 2002; 288(10):1265–8.
6. Prentice AM, Jebb SA. Obesity in Britain: gluttony or sloth? BMJ 1995;311(7002):437–9.
7. Bray G. Health hazards associated with obesity in adults. Available at: http://www.uptodate.com/online/content/topic.do?topicKey=obesity/2127&selected Title=6%7E150&source=search_result. Accessed March 12, 2010.
8. Costigan W, Thordarson D, Debnath U. Operative management of ankle fractures in patients with diabetes mellitus. Foot Ankle Int 2007;28(1):32–7.
9. Flynn JM, Rio FR, Piz PA. Closed ankle fractures in the diabetic patient. Foot Ankle Int 2000;21(4):311–9.
10. Jones KB, Maiers-Yelden KA, Marsh JL, et al. Ankle fractures in patients with diabetes mellitus. J Bone Joint Surg Br 2005;87(4):489–95.
11. White CB, Turner NS, Lee GC, et al. Open ankle fractures in patients with diabetes mellitus. Clin Orthop Relat Res 2003;414:37–44.
12. Wukich D, Kline A. The management of ankle fractures in patients with diabetes. J Bone Joint Surg Am 2008;90(7):1570–8.
13. Blotter RH, Connolly E, Wasan A, et al. Acute complications in the operative treatment of isolated ankle fractures in patients with diabetes mellitus. Foot Ankle Int 1999;20(11):687–94.
14. DeLee J, Drez D, Miller MD. DeLee & Drez's orthopaedic sports medicine: principles and practice, vol. 2. 2nd edition. Philadelphia: Saunders; 2003. p. xxviii, 2623, lx.
15. Einhorn TA. Brain, bone, and body mass: fat is beautiful again. J Bone Joint Surg Am 2001;83(12):1782.
16. Clinical guidelines on the identification, evaluation, and treatment of overweight and obesity in adults—the evidence report. National Institutes of Health. Obes Res 1998;6(Suppl 2):51S–209S.
17. Mokdad AH, Ford ES, Bowman BA, et al. Prevalence of obesity, diabetes, and obesity-related health risk factors, 2001. JAMA 2003;289(1):76–9.
18. Flegal KM, Carroll MD, Ogden CL, et al. Prevalence and trends in obesity among US adults, 1999–2008. JAMA 2010;303(3):235–41.
19. Strauss EJ, Frank JB, Walsh M, et al. Does obesity influence the outcome after the operative treatment of ankle fractures? J Bone Joint Surg Br 2007;89 (6):794–8.
20. Kline AJ, Gruen GS, Pape HC, et al. Early complications following the operative treatment of pilon fractures with and without diabetes. Foot Ankle Int 2009;30(11):1042–7.
21. Fracture and dislocation compendium. Orthopaedic trauma association committee for coding and classification. J Orthop Trauma 1996;10(Suppl 1):1–154, v–ix.
22. Spaine LA, Bollen SR. 'The bigger they come…': the relationship between body mass index and severity of ankle fractures. Injury 1996;27(10):687–9.
23. Guss D, Bhattacharyya T. Perioperative management of the obese orthopaedic patient. J Am Acad Orthop Surg 2006;14(7):425–32.
24. Schricker T, Carvalho G. Pro: tight perioperative glycemic control. J Cardiothorac Vasc Anesth 2005;19 (5):684–8.

25. Vann M. Perioperative management of ambulatory surgical patients with diabetes mellitus. Curr Opin Anaesthesiol 2009;22(6):718–24.

26. Strauss EJ, Egol KA, Alaia M, et al. The use of retrievable inferior vena cava filters in orthopaedic patients. J Bone Joint Surg Br 2008;90(5):662–7.

27. McKee MD, Waddell JP. Intramedullary nailing of femoral fractures in morbidly obese patients. J Trauma 1994;36(2):208–10.

28. Ogunnaike BO, Jones SB, Jones DB, et al. Anesthetic considerations for bariatric surgery. Anesth Analg 2002;95(6):1793–805.

29. Holtom PD. Antibiotic prophylaxis: current recommendations. J Am Acad Orthop Surg 2006;14(10 Spec No.):S98–100.

30. Paiement GD, Renaud E, Dagenais G, et al. Double-blind randomized prospective study of the efficacy of antibiotic prophylaxis for open reduction and internal fixation of closed ankle fractures. J Orthop Trauma 1994;8(1):64–6.

31. Prokuski L. Prophylactic antibiotics in orthopaedic surgery. J Am Acad Orthop Surg 2008;16(5):283–93.

32. Marks RM. Complications of foot and ankle surgery in patients with diabetes. Clin Orthop Relat Res 2001;391:153–61.

33. Jupiter JB, Ring D, Rosen H. The complications and difficulties of management of nonunion in the severely obese. J Orthop Trauma 1995;9(5):363–70.

34. Bstman OM. Body-weight related to loss of reduction of fractures of the distal tibia and ankle. J Bone Joint Surg Br 1995;77(1):101–3.

35. Loder RT. The influence of diabetes mellitus on the healing of closed fractures. Clin Orthop Relat Res 1988;232:210–6.

36. Gandhi A, Doumas C, O'Connor JP, et al. The effects of local platelet rich plasma delivery on diabetic fracture healing. Bone 2006;38(4):540–6.

37. Relwani J, Lahoti O, Orakwe S. Ilizarov ring fixator for a difficult case of ankle syndesmosis disruption. J Foot Ankle Surg 2002;41(5):335–7.

38. Wilson J, Clark J. Obesity: impediment to postsurgical wound healing. Adv Skin Wound Care 2004;17(8):426–35.

39. Abidi NA, Dhawan S, Gruen GS, et al. Wound-healing risk factors after open reduction and internal fixation of calcaneal fractures. Foot Ankle Int 1998;19(12):856–61.

40. Derzie AJ, Silvestri F, Liriano E, et al. Wound closure technique and acute wound complications in gastric surgery for morbid obesity: a prospective randomized trial. J Am Coll Surg 2000;191(3):238–43.

41. Hopf HW, Hunt TK, West JM, et al. Wound tissue oxygen tension predicts the risk of wound infection in surgical patients. Arch Surg 1997;132(9):997–1004 [discussion: 1005].

42. Dietz U, Kuhfuss I, Debus ES, et al. Mario Donati and the vertical mattress suture of the skin. World J Surg 2006;30(2):141–8.

43. Choban PS, Weireter LJ, Maynes C. Obesity and increased mortality in blunt trauma. J Trauma 1991;31(9):1253–7.

44. Timm N, Grupp-Phelan J, Ho M. Chronic ankle morbidity in obese children following an acute ankle injury. Arch Pediatr Adolesc Med 2005;159(1):33–6.

Percutaneous Treatment of Pelvic and Acetabular Fractures in Obese Patients

Peter Bates, FRCS(Orth)[a], Joshua Gary, MD[b],
Gurpreet Singh, MD[b], Charles Reinert, MD[b],
Adam Starr, MD[b],*

KEYWORDS

• Percutaneous • Acetabulum • Pelvic ring • Fractures

Defined as a body mass index (BMI) greater than 30, calculated as the weight in kilograms to the height in meters squared, obesity in the United States is becoming increasingly common. Data from the National Health and Nutrition Examination Survey obtained in 2007 to 2008 showed that 33.8% of the adult population was obese.[1] The steady increase in this population over 20 years has been described as an epidemic,[2] although recent data suggest that the rate of increase appears to be slowing, both in adults and children.[1,3] The implications of this expanding obese population for the trauma orthopedic community are enormous because this population is a discreet group that has a different physiology from the general adult population. Obese patients have higher rates of preexisting comorbidities; their metabolic response to trauma is different and they have higher rates of perioperative complications, such as wound sepsis and venous thromboembolism.[4-7] In addition, there is evidence to suggest that the obese population is at a greater risk of pelvic injuries than the general population.[8]

Through multiple studies, surgical treatment of fractures involving the pelvis and acetabulum has been shown to carry a much greater morbidity when performed in obese patients.[9-13] For pelvic ring injuries, overall complication rates of surgery have been reported to be as high as 54%, with wound sepsis being by far the biggest component.[10] In the acetabulum, rates of wound infection, thromboembolism, and operative blood loss are also increased 2-fold, and these rates follow a linear relationship with body mass, with overall complication rates reaching as high as 63% in morbidly obese patients (BMI>40).[9,13]

With such a bloodcurdling complication profile from traditional surgery, a less-invasive surgical option for these challenging fractures in this high-risk population is potentially very attractive. If the infection rate alone could be reduced, without altering functional outcome, it would yield a huge benefit. For more than 10 years at our institution, we have been percutaneously treating all pelvic ring injuries and many of the acetabular fractures, particularly in high-risk patients, such as those who are obese.

In this article, we present a small consecutive series over 14 months on obese patients who underwent percutaneous treatment of their pelvic or acetabular fractures.

PATIENTS AND METHODS

A retrospective review was performed using our hospital surgical database, after institutional review board approval. Over a 14-month period, between January 2008 and March 2009, the authors performed pelvic or acetabular surgery

[a] Barts and the London NHS trust, Whitechapel, London, E1 1BB, UK
[b] Department of Orthopaedic Surgery, UT Southwestern Medical Center, Dallas, Texas, 5323 Harry Hines Boulevard, Dallas, TX 75390, USA
* Corresponding author.
E-mail address: adam.starr@utsouthwestern.edu

Orthop Clin N Am 42 (2011) 55–67
doi:10.1016/j.ocl.2010.08.004

on 117 consecutive patients. A chart review of each of these surgeries revealed a calculated BMI of 30 or more in 38 patients. Height and weight data were unavailable in one patient, but no other history of obesity was noted in their chart. Of the 38 obese patients, 24 had a pelvic ring injury, 17 had an acetabular fracture, and 3 had a combination of both. Overall, the authors treated 16 pelvic ring injuries and 7 acetabular fractures using percutaneous techniques, making a total of 23 fractures in 20 patients. The fracture types are summarized in **Table 1**. Full medical records were available for review in all 20 patients.

The mean age of the 20 patients was 35 and the average BMI was also 35, with only one patient exceeding the threshold of 40 for being morbidly obese (discussed later in Case Example: Patient 14). There were 14 men and 6 women. Pelvic ring injuries were classified using the system of Young and colleagues[14] and acetabular fractures by that of Letournel and Judet.[15]

Primary outcome measures were postoperative complications requiring repeat surgery, wound infection, deep vein thrombosis (DVT), pulmonary embolus (PE), and radiographic appearance both immediately postoperatively and at follow-up. Deep wound infections were defined as those requiring surgical debridement.

Radiographic Review

Patients with pelvic ring injuries underwent antero-posterior (AP), inlet, and outlet views on admission and at each follow-up, whereas those with acetabular fractures had AP and Judet views. Fracture displacement was measured using pixel calibration with a standard ruler from the Picture Archive Communication System (PACS-MagicWeb, Siemens Inc, New York, New York, USA). Measurements were performed by 2 independent observers (P. B. and J. G.) and a mean calculated. Where multiple views were available, measures showing maximal displacement were chosen.

For the pelvic ring, the method the authors used for measuring displacement was the same as that by LeFaivre and colleagues.[16] A horizontal line is drawn across the superior end plate of the fifth lumbar vertebra. By using this line as a reference from which to make either horizontal measurements (in-line) or vertical ones (perpendicular),

Table 1
Summary of injuries in obese patients and their treatment

Pelvic Ring	Anterior Plating Only	Percutaneous ± Anterior Plating
APC-2	5	4
APC-3	—	6
LC-2	—	2
LC-3	—	2
Vertical Shear	—	2
Jumpers Fracture	—	—
Total	5	16
Open Fractures	—	1
Acetabulum and Pelvis	—	3
Acetabulum	**Open**	**Percutaneous**
Posterior Wall	—	—
Posterior Column	—	—
Anterior Wall	—	—
Anterior Column	—	—
Transverse	—	1
Transverse Posterior Wall	4	2
Posterior Column, Posterior Wall	4	—
T-Type	1	1
Anterior Column, Posterior Hemitransvserse	—	—
Associated Both Column	1	3
Total	10	7

Abbreviations: APC, anteroposterior compression; LC, lateral compression.

the maximum displacement of the anterior and posterior ring could be measured. Displacements were calculated by comparing normal bony landmarks to either the reference line or a perpendicular to it. When there were both pelvic ring and acetabular fractures, bony landmarks that were not involved with the hip injury and whose position was fixed to the constant fragment of the ilium were chosen. The reduction postoperatively and at latest follow-up was recorded and graded according to the method of Tornetta and Matta,[17] with excellent grade being a residual displacement of 0 to 4 mm; good, 4 to 10 mm; fair, 10 to 20 mm; and poor, greater than 20 mm.

For the acetabular fractures, choosing a grading system was more difficult. The authors used the system of Anderson and colleagues,[18] recently described for the assessment of femoral head medialization after a modified Stoppa approach. This approach involves taking a line from the spinous process of L5 down to the symphysis pubis and measuring the difference in the distance between this line and the center of the femoral head on each side. We have graded this as good (0–4 mm), fair (4–10 mm), and poor (greater than 10 mm). Our second outcome was radiological signs of arthritic change at final follow-up, graded 1 to 4 (1, normal appearance; 2, osteophytes; 3, narrowed joint space; 4, bone on bone).

Surgical Technique

General considerations
For both the pelvic ring and acetabulum, patients were positioned supine on a radiolucent bed with the abdomen and ipsilateral lower extremity prepped free. The weight limit of the operating room table was checked in supermorbidly obese patients, and nitrous oxide was avoided with anesthesia because excessive bowel gas can limit fluoroscopic visualization. Intra-abdominal contrast was flushed out where possible. Patients were paralyzed during surgery. Postoperatively, patients were restricted to 3 months of toe-touch—weight bearing on the side of the pelvic ring injury or acetabular fracture.

Pelvic ring
The technique we used for percutaneous pelvic ring fixation has been well documented in the past[16,19] and involves the use of a pelvic reduction frame. (**Fig. 1**) In short, this system enables one side of the pelvis to be stabilized to the operating table, while the other can be manipulated and fine-tuned with a high degree of radiological accuracy and control. One of the strengths of this system is that it allows near-anatomic reductions of the pelvic ring, without the need for either

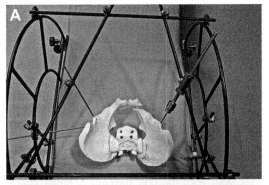

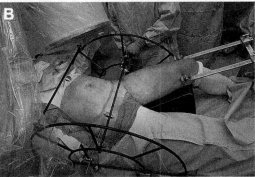

Fig. 1. (*A*) Image of the pelvic reduction frame that allows for closed manipulation of pelvic ring injuries. (*B*) Clinical image demonstrating the use of the Starr Frame. The frame has been anchored to the right hemipelvis. Distal femoral skeletal traction was used on the left femur to assist with closed reduction of the displaced left hemipelvis. Note how the frame allows for appropriate C-arm positioning. (*Courtesy of* Starr Frame LLC, Richardson, TX.)

open approaches or multiple assistants. Our standard fixation was with transsacral iliosacral screws in both S1 and S2, although this varied according to patient anatomy. For the anterior pelvic ring, the technique of fixation depended on the fracture configuration and the soft tissue envelope. Although some symphyseal disruptions were treated with a standard plate and screws, when soft tissues were poor or the fracture was open, an external fixator was used. In one case, a cerclage wire was used. Pubic ramus fractures were generally treated with column screws in this study.

Acetabulum
Screw pathways for fixing acetabular fractures are well described in the literature[20] and are not discussed here. Reduction maneuvers can be divided into closed and open techniques. In any periarticular fracture, there are usually some capsular attachments to the joint fragments, which remain intact after the injury. If patients can be bought to the operating room within a few hours of their

accident, simple fracture patterns such as transverse configurations can be reduced by manipulation of the hip. The most commonly used, of course, is in-line traction, but forced internal or external rotation, flexion, and abduction are all maneuvers that have yielded anatomic reductions for us. Clearly, as time passes, these closed reduction maneuvers become increasingly unlikely to work and most displaced acetabular fractures require some form of open reduction with mini incision.

With the hip flexed up, we perform open reductions with mini incision through a small lateral window, approximately 1 to 2 cm behind the anterior superior iliac crest. A 3- to 5-cm incision is made, and after sharply dissecting off the oblique abdominal wall muscle attachment to the crest, a Cobb elevator can be passed down the inner table directly onto the fracture fragments. In high juxta- and transtectal injuries, the fracture lines can be directly palpated with a finger through the mini lateral window, which gives an additional reading for reduction over fluoroscopy alone. Specialized pelvic reduction clamps have been designed and developed by Charles Reinert, which have sufficient excursion to allow clamping of fractures around voluminous soft tissue envelopes (**Fig. 2**). These clamps allow for transverse fractures to be rotated and compressed, for a displaced dome fragment to be squeezed back down, and for quadrilateral plate medialization to be keyed in. The combination of traction, specific manipulation, and percutaneous clamps allows us to achieve fluoroscopically excellent reductions in most of these cases. If we think that an excellent reduction cannot be achieved minimally invasively, we treat these injuries with open internal fixation via well-described approaches.[21,22] We should also stress that this approach is not straightforward surgery, particularly in those who are obese, and is a technique that has evolved at our institution over the last 10 to 15 years. Each fracture pattern is unique and requires a slightly different screw configuration and reduction maneuver. We advise surgeons who are keen to try this technique to begin with simple, less-displaced fracture patterns before moving on to more complex ones.

Once an acceptable reduction is obtained, the fracture is stabilized with large fragment 6.5-mm or 7.3-mm cannulated screws. The choice of screw pathways is specific to the fracture configuration.

Statistical Analysis

All statistical tests were tabulated using SAS JMP v7 software (SAS Institute Inc, Cary, NC, USA). A

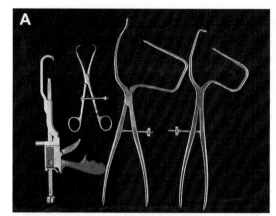
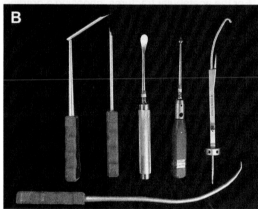

Fig. 2. (*A, B*) Pictures of clamps and other manipulative devices created for percutaneous management of pelvic ring injuries and acetabular fractures. (*Courtesy of* Starr Frame LLC, Richardson, TX.)

Student t-test was used to compare means of continuous variables. Statistical significance was set at a P value of less than .05.

RESULTS
Pelvic Ring

The 16 pelvic fractures had a mean follow-up of 9.7 months (3–24), and there were no deaths. One patient requested to be transferred out of state postoperatively and was subsequently lost to follow-up. The mean initial displacement of the fractures was 22 mm, and final reduction was good or excellent in 15 of the 16 patients, with 7 having a displacement of 4 mm or less. None of the fractures went down by a reduction grade between postoperative and follow-up radiographs. There was a highly significant difference between initial and postoperative displacement ($P = .0007$) but not between the postoperative and final displacement ($P = .54$). Pelvic ring results are summarized in **Table 2**.

Table 2
Pelvic ring injuries: summary of results

Patient	Age (y)	Sex	BMI	Follow-Up Time (mo)	Fracture Type	Initial Displacement (mm)	Postoperative Displacement (mm)	Final Displacement (mm)	Final Grade
1	49	M	31	3	APC-2 (open)	18	7	9	Good
2	19	M	31	4	APC-3	10	3	2	Excellent
3	47	F	31	15	APC-2	7	3	4	Excellent
4	16	M	33	14	APC-3 (bilateral)	6	4	4	Excellent
5	33	M	33	3	LC-3	4	2	2	Excellent
6	34	M	34	8	APC-3	70	8	6	Good
7	62	M	35	9	APC-3	22	2	2	Excellent
8	26	F	36	7	LC-3	15	6	8	Good
9	46	M	32	Lost to follow-up	Vertical shear	47	8	8	Good
10	16	F	34	24	LC-2	13	3	4	Excellent
11	30	M	34	19	APC-3	38	5	5	Good
12	49	M	36	8	APC-3	17	2	2	Excellent
13	67	F	37	9	LC-2 (bilateral)	15	11	16	Fair
14	21	F	45	7	APC-2 (bilateral)	40	7	8	Good
15	25	M	39	8	APC-2	12	5	6	Good
16	16	M	36	8	Vertical shear	22	7	8	Good
Mean	35	—	35	9.7	—	22	5	5.3	—

Abbreviations: F, female; LC, lateral compression; M, male.

Complications

There were no infections in this group, either superficial or deep, and there were no postoperative DVTs or PEs. Three patients, in whom adequate prophylaxis was impossible, received temporary central venous filters, but all 3 filters were subsequently removed. There were no new postoperative neurologic deficits. There were 2 scheduled returns to the operating theater, for supplementary anterior fixation. One of these (patient 6) patients was a 34-year-old man with a severe AP compression (APC) type 3 injury. Having stabilized his pelvic ring posteriorly, the anterior plating was postponed by 2 weeks because of an open laparotomy wound, which extended very distally. Once his soft tissues were more compliant, the symphysis was plated, with no further complications. The second case is reported later in the section Patient 14: Case Example.

The least favorable outcome was observed in a 67-year-old lady (the oldest in this series) with moderately displaced bilateral insufficiency fractures and unilateral ramus fractures after a fall down the steps. Her BMI was 37, and it was thought initially that she could be treated nonoperatively. However, as a result of ongoing pain and further displacement observed on serial radiographs, the patient required surgery at 17 days. Bilateral posterior percutaneous iliosacral screws were passed after closed reduction with the frame, and postoperative radiographs showed some improvement (from 15 to 11 mm of displacement). However, her follow-up radiographs showed that she had "settled" back to the preinjury position. With a displacement of 16 mm at follow-up, the patient's result was graded as "fair."

There were no cases of heterotopic ossification (Brooker grade 2 or worse) on the last follow-up radiographs, but 3 of the 16 patients with pelvic ring injuries did undergo removal of symptomatic hardware after bony union.

Acetabulum

The 7 acetabular fractures treated percutaneously had a mean follow-up of 9.1 months (4–18 months) with none lost to follow-up and no deaths. One patient had an undisplaced, transverse, posterior wall fracture, but all the others were initially displaced with a mean of 17 mm (9–22 mm). Patient data for the acetabular fractures are summarized in **Table 3**.

Complications

There were no infections in this group, either superficial or deep, and no cases of postoperative DVTs or PEs. One patient (described later in Case

Example: Patient 14) made a scheduled return to surgery for supplementary anterior fixation of her pelvic ring, but there were no other returns to the operating theater acutely. There were no new postoperative neurologic deficits, and none of the patients had developed heterotopic ossification (Brooker grade 2 or worse) at their latest follow-up. Immediate postoperative reduction was graded "good" in all cases, but there was a loss of reduction and subsequent development of arthritis (grade 4) in 2 of the 7 cases requiring total hip replacement (patients 17 and 19). Aged 51 and 71 years, these patients were at the older end of our group, and both patients had complex fracture patterns (T-type and associated both column) in relatively osteopenic bone with large preoperative medialization of the head (22 and 15 mm). In both patients, the initial postoperative position was good, with minimal medialization (2 mm in both), no articular step, and no visible articular gapping larger than 1 to 2 mm on any of the 3 views. Both had failure of fixation between 2 and 4 weeks and were reported in the chart as having been partially weight bearing. By this time it was thought that these patients would be better served by delayed hip arthroplasty rather than revision fixation, and both have done well after their hip replacements.

Discounting the undisplaced fracture, for the 6 displaced acetabular fractures, we had 2 failures of fixation, making an overall complication rate of 33%.

Case Example: Patient 14

The patient was a 21-year-old pedestrian who was struck by a car. She sustained bilateral APC injuries, along with bilateral transverse acetabular fractures, displaced on the right and undisplaced on the left (**Figs. 3–5**). The patient was morbidly obese, with a BMI of 45 (the largest of our series). After applying traction and a binder in the emergency room, she was taken to surgery on the day of injury and the displaced acetabular fracture was managed initially. Through a 5-cm lateral window and with the hip flexed, a minimally invasive collinear clamp was passed down the inner table, into the lesser notch. With traction and deployment of the clamp, the fracture was reduced. This reduction was confirmed both by direct palpation with a finger down the inner table and by multiplanar fluoroscopy. The fracture was reduced and stabilized in the standard fashion, with anterior and posterior column screws (6.5 mm cannulated).

The pelvic ring was then reduced using the reduction frame. Initially, the left (least unstable)

Table 3
Acetabular fractures: summary of results

Patient	Age (y)	Sex	BMI	Follow-Up (mo)	Fracture Type	Type of Fixation	Preoperative Displacement	Postoperative Displacement	Follow-Up Displacement
14	21	F	45	4	Transverse	ACS	17	1	1
15	25	M	39	8	Transverse posterior wall	ACS	9	2	3
16	18	M	36	11	Associated both column	ACS/LC-2	20	1	1
17[a]	51	M	31	7	Associated both column	LC-2/Magic	15	2	12
18	59	F	34	18	Associated both column	LC-2/LC-2	18	8	8
19[a]	71	M	35	8	T-type	LC-2/Magic/SAS x2	22	2	13
20	24	M	37	8	Transverse posterior wall (undisplaced)	ACS	0	0	0
Mean	38.4	—	36.7	9.1	—	—	14.4	2.3	5.4

Abbreviations: ACS, anterior column screw; F, female; LC-2, LC-2 screw; Magic, magic screw; M, male; SAS, supra-acetabular screw.
[a] Failure of fixation between 2 and 4 weeks.

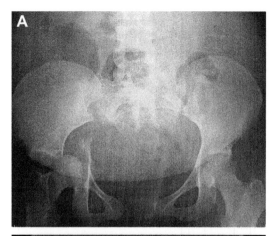

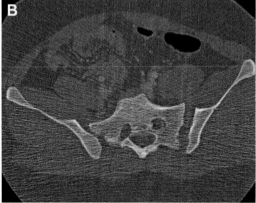

Fig. 3. (A) Preoperative AP pelvis and (B) axial computed tomographic scan showing a displaced transverse right acetabular fracture and bilateral APC pelvic ring injuries in a 21-year-old woman.

side was reduced and then fixed using an S2 iliosacral screw going into the sacral body. The left side was then stabilized to the frame and the right side reduced onto it, using the frame elements. Once a good reduction was achieved, final definitive fixation was placed with a single transsacral S1 screw and bilateral S2 screws (all were 7.3 mm). At this point it was noted that the patient had a residual symphyseal diastasis, which could be only partially controlled by an external fixator. It was thought that she was too unstable to tolerate further surgery, and therefore, her symphyseal fixation was postponed by 5 days. Through a Pfannenstiel approach, the symphysis was exposed but could not be plated because of the narrow ramus being completely filled by a 6.5-mm screw. The diastasis was therefore cabled together, using a cable passer through the obturator foramen under direct vision.

There was some residual widening of 7 mm of the right sacroiliac joint after this procedure, which remained largely unchanged at final follow-up. For

both acetabulum and pelvic ring, the patient was graded as "good" and she had an otherwise uncomplicated follow-up. At latest follow-up the patient had symmetric pain-free hip movements and was walking without aids. There was no evidence of early hip arthritis, but she was complaining of some mild back symptoms.

DISCUSSION

Pelvic ring injuries and acetabular fractures are severe injuries, which are commonly treated with reduction and internal fixation via large surgical approaches. Complications occur in the best hands, but with the obese population, they have been shown to increase sharply, in an almost linear fashion with the size of the patient.[9] Of the reported complications, infection and wound breakdown are by far the most common.

For the pelvic ring, Sems and colleagues[10] recently described their experience of treating pelvic fractures in 48 obese patients, comparing their outcomes to a larger cohort of 134 patients who were not obese. The investigators found that complication rates in obese patients were 54% compared with 15% in those who were not obese. They found not only significantly higher wound complications in the obese group (25%) compared with the nonobese group (5.9%) but also a significantly greater rate of loss of reduction (31% vs 6%). The investigators stipulate clearly that all the infections and wound problems occurred around open exposures. There were no infections in the 18 patients receiving only percutaneous surgery. This mirrors our findings from the 16 pelvic ring injuries described in this article in which none of the patients developed infections. Of those 16 patients, 4 underwent symphyseal plating through a Pfannenstiel approach as part of their fixation. We have included these cases in our percutaneous cohort because the reduction was all done closed and the posterior pelvic ring was universally treated with iliosacral screws alone. Sems and colleagues noted a 14% infection rate with anterior plating of the symphysis; in our small series of 4, there were no infections, although 2 were delayed because of either noncompliant soft tissues or anesthetic issues.

Sems and colleagues also found that loss of reduction was clearly a problem in the obese patients (31% in obese patients vs 6% in nonobese patients), particularly in the Orthopaedic Trauma Association type C injuries. However, the investigators were unable to comment on whether there was a difference between the percutaneous group and the open surgical group in terms of reduction loss, so it is unclear whether open reduction of

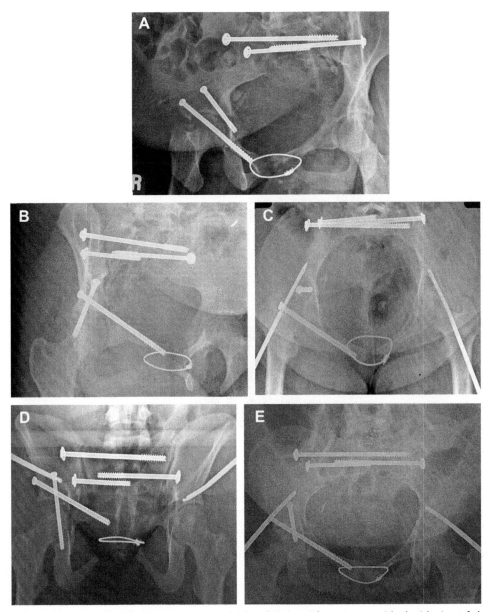

Fig. 4. (*A*) Postoperative AP, (*B*) inlet, (*C*) outlet, and (*D*) Judet views show some residual widening of the right sacroiliac joint, (*E*) but an otherwise well-aligned pelvic ring and acetabulum.

the posterior pelvis conferred any significant benefit in terms of stability. We noted one loss of position between the time of surgery and follow-up (patient 13) making a complication rate of 6%. Our previously reported experience of percutaneous pelvic ring fixation has also shown loss of position rates to be comparable with the reported outcomes of open reductions.[16] Since the findings of Griffin and colleagues,[23] who found a 13% failure rate of unilateral iliosacral screws in vertically unstable sacral fractures, we have changed our posterior fixation to transsacral screws, which pass right through the sacrum and anchor in the tricortical bone of the sacral ala and opposing ilium. Anecdotally, since making this change, our failure rates in vertically unstable fractures have decreased and we feel that this series reflects that.

Porter and colleagues[12] recently published a study similarly designed to that of Sems and colleague. They compared 186 nonobese patients with 102 obese ones. In terms of wound complications, the obese group was at much greater risk, with a 39% incidence compared with 19% in the nonobese group. Failures of fixation were

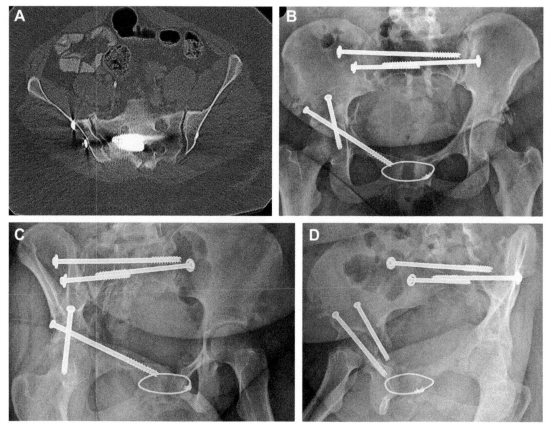

Fig. 5. (*A–D*) Radiographs at 4-months follow-up confirm that the sacroiliac alignment has not changed and the acetabulum shows no signs of arthrosis.

approximately equal between the 2 groups, running at around 7%. This finding is more in keeping with Lefaivre and colleagues'[16] recent article in which no correlation was found between obesity and final quality of reduction.

For the acetabulum, complication rates after open surgery range from 38% to 63% across different studies.[13,24] BMI and complication rates appear to have a linear relationship, with statistically significant increases in operative time, hospital stay, and blood loss reported in morbidly obese patients.[13] Naturally, there are several technical difficulties associated with performing complex acetabular reconstructions in obese patients. The surgical approaches are usually more difficult, requiring longer deeper incisions to achieve adequate visualization. Standard pelvic instrumentation may be difficult to apply around the excessive envelope, and the sheer volume of soft tissue can make preoperative and intraoperative imaging very difficult to interpret. Porter and colleagues recently stated, "…operative fixation of displaced acetabular fractures in the morbidly obese population may possess a complication

rate that outweighs the potential for a successful outcome."

Percutaneous management of undisplaced acetabular fractures is well described by several authors and commonly practiced to improve pain and prevent displacement in certain fracture types.[25,26] Percutaneous treatment of displaced fractures remains controversial, with only 1 previous report in the literature.[27] In the obese population, a minimally invasive option offers several advantages, including shorter operation times, minimal incisions, negligible blood loss, and very low infection rates. However, not all acetabular fracture types are amenable to percutaneous fixation, and in our institution, those fractures that are not amenable are treated with standard open techniques via well-described extensile approaches.[21,22] Undisplaced and minimally displaced fractures in this population are typically treated percutaneously. Displaced transverse fractures and those involving the anterior column are also suitable for minimally invasive surgery if an excellent reduction can be achieved. However, displaced fractures of the posterior wall and posterior column, along with T-type variants with posterior displacement are not considered candidates for this type of surgery.

In this study we have presented 7 acetabular fractures, 6 of which were displaced. Notably, there were no infections, no deaths, no neurologic injuries, and no cases of proven DVT or PE. At follow-up, there were no cases of heterotopic ossification requiring excision, and none required hardware removal.

Much of the publicly expressed concern around the percutaneous treatment of acetabular fractures has been the ability to both achieve an anatomic reduction and to maintain it. In our series, all of the fractures had good reductions immediately postoperatively, with minimal medialization and good articular congruity. However, 2 of the fractures (33% of the initially displaced ones) did displace between 2 and 6 weeks with negative consequences for the hip joint. Both of these patients were older than the mean (aged 51 and 71 years), with osteoporotic fracture configurations and may have had some compliance issues, all of which may have contributed to the failure.

In Porter and colleagues'[13] recent study, they reported a 10% loss of fixation in the obese group that was studied, which is clearly superior to our small series. However, this loss of fixation has to be counterbalanced by their 46% wound complication rate, the 5% of nerve injuries, and 3 deaths, not to mention the 5% of patients requiring excision of heterotopic ossification and 15% requiring removal of hardware. Mayo reported an obese subset of 21 patients from a cohort of 105. He reported a complication rate of 38%, which was mainly populated by infections and wound problems (24%), with failure of fixation in 5%.[24]

Russell and colleagues[11] described several unusual complications in their series of 12 overweight and 5 obese patients, as part of a much larger cohort of 131 acetabular fractures treated with open surgery. Of the complications, 24% were related to positioning of the patients, and a further 24% developed wound breakdown. Loss of fixation in the entire cohort was only seen in 2 early ambulators.

Our series contrasts strongly with these other studies. Excluding the one undisplaced fracture, our overall complication rate was 33%, composed of the 2 fixation failures. We saw no wound problems or infections, no neurologic injuries, no DVTs or PEs, and no problems with heterotopic ossification. Both of our failures of fixation were in older patients with more osteoporotic fracture configurations, and both were reported in their charts to have walked on their fixation early. Nonetheless, it would seem that percutaneously fixed acetabular fractures are less resistant to early failure than those treated open. The issue is therefore whether we are able to reduce these early failures by either better patient selection or better supervision of postoperative weight-bearing status.

This article has several limitations. It is a retrospective review, with all the inherent shortcomings that come with that. The numbers are small compared with other studies, with only 16 pelvic ring injuries and 7 acetabular fractures, 3 patients being in both groups. It is therefore difficult to raise any meaningful statistical analysis. We also have no control group against which to compare our results. We did treat 10 acetabular fractures in obese patients with open surgery (see **Table 1**), but we did not think that this was a valid control group because these patients had been deemed unsuitable for percutaneous surgery at the time of admission. These patients had a different set of injury types, not amenable to minimally invasive surgery, and we felt that a direct comparison would be misleading. BMI was calculated from height and weight data recorded by the nursing staff in the patients' charts. However, we cannot be certain of whether these indices were formally measured or simply volunteered by the patients, making their accuracy uncertain. Self-reporting of height and weight has been shown to be commonly inaccurate.[28] Our follow-up was short (around 9 months) and 1 of the patients with pelvic ring injuries was lost to follow-up. However, all the injuries had united by the time of their last appointment.

Radiological end points remain a problem for both pelvic and acetabular fractures. Radiographs are rarely of identical rotation and viewing angle, which makes for potential errors in measurement. For the acetabulum, applying the classical grading system of Matta[29] after percutaneous treatment is problematic because it emphasizes reduction of both the columns and the articular surface. Percutaneous fixation with 6.5-mm screws usually obscures the visible joint line on at least 2 views, making this an unreliable parameter. Also, when treated percutaneously, the quadrilateral plate often remains medially displaced, despite the dome fragment and the head being reduced. We therefore used radiological parameters that can be reliably measured and that correlate with functional outcome.

Another limitation is that percutaneous techniques have evolved over time at our institution, with the whole surgical team completely familiar with the surgery. Translating this procedure to another center might not deliver the same results, particularly in the short term. On the positive side, all surgeries were performed by the same 2 surgeons, with a common pre- and postoperative management protocol and rehabilitation schedule.

Overall, this study is limited in several ways, particularly by size, but the outcomes of our small cohort of patients are so contrasting with the historical literature, we feel that it is worthy of reporting. It is also, to our knowledge, the first description of percutaneous acetabular fracture fixation being used in an obese population.

SUMMARY

We believe that with careful patient selection, percutaneous treatment of acetabular fractures is a good alternative to traditional open management in high-risk patient groups, such as those who are obese. For pelvic ring injuries, the reduction frame is an effective way of achieving bony alignment of each hemipelvis, regardless of patient size. We have found that percutaneous stabilization has not resulted in a tendency to loose reduction. With only 1 fixation failure in this series and no reported complications, we believe that percutaneous treatment of pelvic ring injuries in the obese population is a compelling alternative to open surgery.

REFERENCES

1. Flegal KM, Carroll MD, Ogden CL, et al. Prevalence and trends in obesity among US adults, 1999–2008. JAMA 2010;303(3):235–41.
2. Wyatt SB, Winters KP, Dubbert PM. Overweight and obesity: prevalence, consequences, and causes of a growing public health problem. Am J Med Sci 2006;331(4):166–74.
3. Ogden CL, Carroll MD, Curtin LR, et al. Prevalence of high body mass index in US children and adolescents, 2007–2008. JAMA 2010;303(3):242–9.
4. Guss D, Bhattacharyya T. Perioperative management of the obese orthopaedic patient. J Am Acad Orthop Surg 2006;14(7):425–32.
5. Brown CV, Neville AL, Rhee P, et al. The impact of obesity on the outcomes of 1153 critically injured blunt trauma patients. J Trauma 2005;59(5): 1048–51 [discussion: 51].
6. Choban PS, Weireter LJ Jr, Maynes C. Obesity and increased mortality in blunt trauma. J Trauma 1991;31(9):1253–7.
7. Bochicchio GV, Joshi M, Bochicchio K, et al. Impact of obesity in the critically ill trauma patient: a prospective study. J Am Coll Surg 2006;203(4):533–8.
8. Boulanger BR, Milzman D, Mitchell K, et al. Body habitus as a predictor of injury pattern after blunt trauma. J Trauma 1992;33(2):228–32.
9. Karunakar MA, Shah SN, Jerabek S. Body mass index as a predictor of complications after operative treatment of acetabular fractures. J Bone Joint Surg Am 2005;87(7):1498–502.
10. Sems SA, Johnson M, Cole PA, et al. Elevated body mass index increases early complications of surgical treatment of pelvic ring injuries. J Orthop Trauma 2010;24(5):309–14.
11. Russell GV Jr, Nork SE, Chip Routt ML Jr. Perioperative complications associated with operative treatment of acetabular fractures. J Trauma 2001;51(6): 1098–103.
12. Porter SE, Graves ML, Qin Z, et al. Operative experience of pelvic fractures in the obese. Obes Surg 2008;18(6):702–8.
13. Porter SE, Russell GV, Dews RC, et al. Complications of acetabular fracture surgery in morbidly obese patients. J Orthop Trauma 2008;22(9): 589–94.
14. Young JW, Burgess AR, Brumback RJ, et al. Pelvic fractures: value of plain radiography in early assessment and management. Radiology 1986;160(2): 445–51.
15. Letournel E, Judet R. Fractures of the acetabulum. In: Elson RA, editor. Berlin (Heidelburg): Springer-Verlag; 1981.
16. Lefaivre KA, Starr AJ, Barker BP, et al. Early experience with reduction of displaced disruption of the pelvic ring using a pelvic reduction frame. J Bone Joint Surg Br 2009;91(9):1201–7.
17. Tornetta P 3rd, Matta JM. Outcome of operatively treated unstable posterior pelvic ring disruptions. Clin Orthop Relat Res 1996;329:186–93.
18. Andersen RC, O'Toole RV, Nascone JW, et al. Modified Stoppa approach for acetabular fractures with anterior and posterior column displacement: quantification of radiographic reduction and analysis of interobserver variability. J Orthop Trauma 2010; 24(5):271–8.
19. Lefaivre KA, Starr AJ, Reinert CM. Reduction of displaced pelvic ring disruptions using a pelvic reduction frame. J Orthop Trauma 2009;23(4): 299–308.
20. Tile M, Helfet DL, Kellam JF. Fractures of the pelvis and acetabulum. 3rd edition. Lipincott Williams and Wilkins.
21. Reinert CM, Bosse MJ, Poka A, et al. A modified extensile exposure for the treatment of complex or malunited acetabular fractures. J Bone Joint Surg Am 1988;70(3):329–37.
22. Lefaivre KA, Starr AJ, Reinert CM. A modified anterior exposure to the acetabulum for treatment of difficult anterior acetabular fractures. J Orthop Trauma 2009;23(5):370–8.
23. Griffin DR, Starr AJ, Reinert CM, et al. Vertically unstable pelvic fractures fixed with percutaneous iliosacral screws: does posterior injury pattern predict fixation failure? J Orthop Trauma 2003; 17(6):399–405.

24. Mayo KA. Open reduction and internal fixation of fractures of the acetabulum. Results in 163 fractures. Clin Orthop Relat Res 1994;305:31–7.

25. Giannoudis PV, Tzioupis CC, Pape HC, et al. Percutaneous fixation of the pelvic ring: an update. J Bone Joint Surg Br 2007;89(2):145–54.

26. Parker PJ, Copeland C. Percutaneous fluoroscopic screw fixation of acetabular fractures. Injury 1997; 28(9–10):597–600.

27. Starr AJ, Jones AL, Reinert CM, et al. Preliminary results and complications following limited open reduction and percutaneous screw fixation of displaced fractures of the acetabulum. Injury 2001; 32(Suppl 1):SA45–50.

28. Niedhammer I, Bugel I, Bonenfant S, et al. Validity of self-reported weight and height in the French GAZEL cohort. Int J Obes Relat Metab Disord 2000; 24(9):1111–8.

29. Matta JM. Fractures of the acetabulum: accuracy of reduction and clinical results in patients managed operatively within three weeks after the injury. J Bone Joint Surg Am 1996;78(11):1632–45.

Open Treatment of Pelvic and Acetabular Fractures

F. Keith Gettys, MD[a], George V. Russell, MD[b],
Madhav A. Karunakar, MD[a],*

KEYWORDS

• Pelvic fracture • Acetabular fracture • Operative • Obese

Pelvic and acetabular fractures most frequently result from high-energy motor vehicle trauma or falls. Open reduction and internal fixation of these fractures requires an extensive surgical approach that is often associated with long operative times, high blood loss, and a significant risk of postoperative complications. The prevalence of obesity in the United States currently exceeds 25% and is projected to exceed 40% by 2025.[1,2] Recent reports have noted a higher rate of complications after the operative treatment of pelvic and acetabular fractures compared with patients of normal weight.[3–6] This article summarizes the current literature on open treatment of pelvic and acetabular fractures in the obese patient, reviews the physiologic adaptations of obesity as they relate to pelvic surgery, highlights risk factors for complications, and provides recommendations to reduce the incidence of complications.

Once the decision has been made to proceed with operative treatment of a pelvic or acetabular fracture, the method of definitive treatment may need to be modified based on patient factors such as associated injuries, status of the soft tissue in and around the zone of injury, or medical comorbidities. Obesity has been associated with a wide spectrum of comorbidities that affect nearly every organ system, including cardiac, pulmonary, endocrine, and neurologic systems.[7–9] The orthopedic surgeon needs to be aware and understand the altered physiology of an obese patient and that

adjustments may need to be made preoperatively, intraoperatively, and postoperatively in the management of the obese patient with an operative pelvic or acetabular fracture.

INITIAL EVALUATION

The initial assessment and evaluation of a pelvic and acetabular fracture in the patient who is obese is more difficult than for a patient who is not obese. These injuries may result in life-threatening hemorrhage, and prompt recognition of these injuries is critical. Standard advanced trauma life support evaluation and resuscitation protocols should be followed. Fluid resuscitation and the use of blood are critical because the cardiac system of patients who are obese may already be stressed by adaptations made as it attempts to perfuse the increased tissue mass. The orthopedic examination of the pelvis and extremities can be more difficult secondary to the body habitus. A visual inspection should be made for signs of hemorrhage or open wounds. All skin folds, including the panniculi, need to be examined because they can hide wounds. Anterior pelvic injuries should increase suspicion for urethral injuries. Careful inspection of the groin, perineum, buttocks, and posterior pelvis should be performed for possible wounds or blood at the urethral meatus. A speculum examination should be performed in women with anterior pelvic injuries. The increased soft

The authors have nothing to disclose.
[a] Department of Orthopaedic Surgery, Carolinas Medical Center, 1025 Morehead Medical Drive, Suite 300, Charlotte, NC 28204, USA
[b] Department of Orthopaedic Surgery, University of Mississippi, 2500 North State Street, Jackson, MS 39216, USA
* Corresponding author.
E-mail address: madhav.karunakar@carolinashealthcare.org

Orthop Clin N Am 42 (2011) 69–83
doi:10.1016/j.ocl.2010.08.006

tissue can make soft tissue swelling less obvious and bony palpation more difficult. The sensory and motor examination can be more challenging in the obese patient because abnormalities related to diabetes or vascular disease are common.[9] A thorough examination must include palpation and examination of all extremities to identify any other injuries. The morbidly obese patient has a baseline decreased range of motion of the hips, knees, and other joints, so the examiner should be alert to any asymmetries on examination.

Before the definitive treatment plan can be made, a complete radiographic assessment of the pelvis and acetabulum is required. This radiographic evaluation of the obese patient can be more challenging because the increased adipose tissue can lead to inadequate penetration of the x-rays, resulting in increased noise and low image contrast.[10] In addition, an increase in the time required for penetration results in motion artifact, further degrading the quality of plain films. To improve image quality, reacquisition and postacquisition adjustments can be made, including the use of a Bucky grid to minimize scatter, increasing the kilovolts peak and milliamperes to improve penetration and increasing the film development speed.[10]

Computed tomography (CT) is routinely performed in trauma patients to assess for visceral injuries. Bony cuts and reconstructions can be helpful in delineating fracture patterns and for preoperative planning. The weight or size of the obese patient needs to be considered, because it may exceed the limits for the CT scanner available in the hospital. Most institutions have CT scanners with table weight limits of approximately 200 kg and an available gantry diameter limit of 52 to 55 cm.[10] In a recent national survey of hospitals, it was estimated that only 10% of emergency departments and 34% of trauma centers have access to these large weight capacity CT scanners.[11] Veterinary schools and some zoos have access to larger-capacity CT scanners that could theoretically be used.[9]

For some acetabular fractures with an associated posterior dislocation or central protrusion, the femoral head may not remain concentrically reduced under the roof of the acetabulum without skeletal traction. Typically, the amount of weight used for skeletal traction is 1/10 to 1/6 of the patient's body weight (between 10 and 15 kg for a patient weighing 90 kg), which would result in significantly larger amounts of weight in the obese patient. Any larger amount of weight should be applied gradually and with caution because there is an increased risk of soft tissue or nerve injury with higher weights. The larger soft tissue envelope in the obese patient may not allow the standard traction pin to clear the soft tissues, decreasing the working length of the pin, and requiring the use of larger pins. A larger pin can lead to greater soft tissue damage during insertion, further increasing the risk of a pin tract infection. For the largest patients, it has been necessary to use the starting guidewire for a femoral nails to traverse the mass of the lower thigh. Larger tension bows might also be required and, if used, should be adequately padded to prevent compression on the anterior tibial skin, which can lead to skin necrosis or pressure ulcers.

PERIOPERATIVE CONSIDERATIONS

Obesity is an independent risk factor for cardiovascular disease, which increases the risk of perioperative complications.[12–14] The cardiac system of an obese patient has several differences from a patient of normal weight. Morbid obesity is often associated with left ventricular enlargement, systolic and diastolic dysfunction (risk factors for acute ischemia or infarction), congestive heart failure, and sudden death.[15] In addition, hypertension, hyperlipidemia, and diabetes mellitus are more common in the obese and are associated with the development of coronary artery disease.[7] More specifically, the patient who is obese has an increased total blood volume because of the increased requirement from the greater body mass. The cardiac output of obese patients increases proportionally and can be 40% greater than that of patients with normal body weight.[16] Pelvic and acetabular fractures are frequently associated with significant blood loss. This blood loss, combined with preexisting increased work demand, can overload the heart and increase the mortality risk. For this reason, obese patients must be adequately resuscitated before undergoing operative repair and may require the use of invasive hemodynamic monitoring to maintain cardiac index.[17]

In addition to the physiologic adaptations to the cardiac system, the obese patient also experiences alterations to the pulmonary system. Patients who are obese have decreased chest wall compliance because of increased adipose tissue in the abdomen and chest wall.[16] The lung compliance may be only 35% of a patient who is not obese.[16] Also, patients who are obese have inefficient respiratory muscles, with an increased work of breathing. The increased metabolic activity of the excess fat and soft tissue results in greater oxygen consumption and carbon dioxide production.[18] Compared with individuals of normal weight, patients who are obese have greater intra-abdominal pressures, caused by the increased weight, which decreases functional residual capacity, expiratory reserve volume, and total lung capacity.[18,19] The patient who is obese requires more diaphragmatic excursion to have the same ventilation as a patient of normal weight. The changes that are present in an obese patient at baseline are exacerbated when the patient is given anesthesia and positioned for surgery. Obese patients are at increased risk for pulmonary aspiration and pneumonitis because they have higher gastric residual volumes with lower gastric pH.[20] Combining these factors with poor ventilation places the obese patient at higher risk for atelectasis and pneumonia.

Type II diabetes mellitus is strongly associated with obesity, and similarly is an independent risk factor for postoperative complications. Some of the deleterious effects of obesity have been believed to be attributable, at least in part, to derangements in metabolic function.[21] Insulin resistance is a major factor and plays a large role in obesity-related metabolic derangements. The lack of insulin results in hyperglycemia, decreased protein synthesis, increased protein degradation, increased susceptibility to infection, and reduced antiapoptotic (prosurvival) and antiinflammatory actions of insulin.[21–24] The stress response from the trauma and pain during the perioperative period can lead to release of catecholamines that can increase blood glucose levels in patients with or without history of diabetes. This hyperglycemia can negatively effect wound healing by inhibiting the inflammatory response, impairing immunity, and interfering with collagen synthesis.[25] Diabetes mellitus, alone, leads to impaired immune responses with impaired chemotaxis, phagocytosis, and bactericidal ability of the neutrophils, monocytes, and macrophages.[26] Strict perioperative glycemic control has been shown to reduce morbidity and mortality, and to reduce postoperative infections.[15,27,28]

INTRAOPERATIVE CONSIDERATIONS
Patient Positioning

The weight of the patient needs to be considered when determining whether the operating room table will be secure and safe for the patient. Most standard operating room tables have a safe weight limit of 200 to 225 kg, but some manufacturers offer newer operating tables that can accommodate up to 450 kg.[29,30] If the high-capacity table is not available, 2 tables can be secured head to head or side by side. However, this 2-table arrangement can make intraoperative fluoroscopic imaging more difficult. Lifts can be

placed under the table for additional support. Surgical patients who are obese are prone to falling off during positioning, and bean bags and straps should be placed to secure the patient to the table and prevent falls during table position changes.[31]

Because obese patients who have a pelvic or acetabular fracture may present with borderline physiology (as discussed previously), careful consideration of surgical positioning must be made because intraoperative positioning can affect the patient's ability to tolerate the procedure. Although patient positioning is most commonly determined by fracture pattern and surgical approach, the surgeon should recognize that positions that restrict chest and abdominal motion can compromise ventilation and are poorly tolerated by obese patients. The supine and prone positions can result in compression of the vena cava and the aorta as well as compression of the diaphragm, making ventilation more difficult.[16,30] The lateral decubitus is best tolerated by obese patients, because the weight of the panniculus adiposus is off the abdomen, allowing for greater diaphragmatic excursion.[16,32] The lateral position may also allow for posterior soft tissues to fall away, improving access to the acetabulum.

AUTHORS' PREFERRED PRACTICE: PATIENT POSITIONING
Supine Position

Patients are positioned on a radiolucent table on a lumbosacral support placed in the midline of the back from the inferior angle of the scapula distally to the proximal aspect of the anal crease. This position allows for the soft tissues to be elevated off the bed and also allows for the panniculi to fall posteriorly instead of pushing laterally where the exposure is to be made. Rolled sheets or blankets are used to allow for intraoperative fluoroscopic imaging. The chest is stabilized with a padded belt. Another precaution is to securely stabilize the nonoperative extremities, particularly the lower extremities. Because the obese patient is wide compared with the radiolucent table, it is easy for the nonoperative lower extremity to roll off the table. The authors have used Ace wraps over foam padding to secure the lower extremities.

Positioning the abdominal panniculus may prove challenging. If the panniculus is especially large it may have to be secured to provide access to the operative field. The most common method is to tape the panniculus to the opposite side of the table from the operative field (**Fig. 1**). An adhesive is applied to the skin to allow the tape to stick well to the panniculus. The panniculus is then pulled

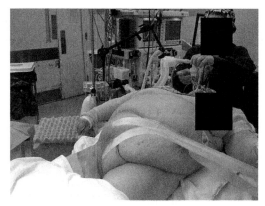

Fig. 1. This patient had a large abdominal panniculus that required taping for access to the groin for an arterial line and eventual exposure to the ilium. (*Courtesy of* George V. Russell, MD.)

Prone Position

Prone positioning is used frequently for stabilization of acetabular fractures and pelvic ring injuries. To avoid difficulties with ventilation in the prone position, it is imperative that the abdomen be allowed to hang free, preventing excessive intra-abdominal pressure that may contribute to ventilatory compromise. Longitudinal chest rolls are typically positioned on each side of the patient from the chest distally to the anterior superior iliac spine. The chest rolls must not be placed distal into the femoral canal because the patient's weight against the roll may result in a femoral nerve palsy. If the patient has a particularly wide panniculus or protuberant abdomen, then transverse rolls are used. One roll is placed transversely across the chest and another transversely across the anterior superior iliac spines. Sheets or blankets are added to the rolls to ensure that the abdomen hangs free and the patient can be adequately ventilated (**Fig. 2**). If the abdomen is markedly obese, then, in addition to transverse chest rolls, the abdomen may need to be folded under to the nonoperative side to allow the surgeon closer access to the operative site (**Fig. 3**).

The knees are especially susceptible to pressure in the prone position and must be protected against pressure necrosis. Donut pads are used beneath the knees to protect the skin over the patellae. The legs are placed on a pillow to prevent the toes from contacting the surgical bed. The nonoperative limb is stabilized with an Ace wrap.

under tension to allow visualization of the proposed operative site. Another method is to sew the panniculus with large sutures to the chest wall. This method obviates concern about losing adhesion of tape. When using these techniques, the authors recommend that the patient's ventilatory status should be observed before initiating surgery, because the extra weight of the abdomen on the chest may obstruct ventilation of the patient, necessitating release of the pannicular strapping.

If pannicular strapping is not possible, one may take advantage of the mobile nature of the panniculus. The panniculus may be gently placed or rocked away from the operative field. The weight of the abdomen will often keep much of the panniculus away from the operative field. Although not as effective as pannicular strapping, this method allows for improved visualization. Rotating the surgical table away from the surgeon is an option, but patients who are obese are much more prone to roll off the table than patients who are lean.

Lateral Position

Positioning devices or beanbags may be used to secure a patient in the lateral position. The authors prefer beanbags to positioning devises for better control of the abdomen. An extra-large beanbag is often required, but on the most obese patients, 2 beanbags taped together may be required

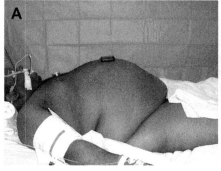
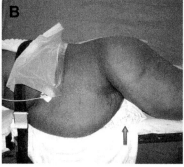

Fig. 2. (*A*) This morbidly obese patient had a remarkably large abdomen. A pager was placed on his abdomen for scale. (*B*) In the prone position, transverse rolls (*arrow*) were required to allow for adequate pressure release on his abdomen. (*Courtesy of* George V. Russell, MD.)

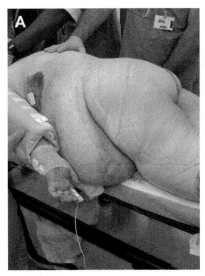
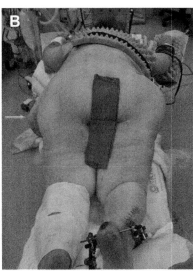

Fig. 3. (*A*) This patient had a large abdominal panniculus that required folding the panniculus underneath the patient to the side opposite surgery. (*B*) The same patient as noted in (*A*), viewed from the foot of the bed. The patient had large buttock/thigh folds bilaterally. Note the extra fold on the left side (*arrow*), which is the abdominal panniculus that has been folded under the patient, away from the proposed operative hip on the right side. Also note the pressure sore on the patient's right heel. (*Courtesy of* George V. Russell, MD.)

(**Fig. 4**). A positioning pillow originally designed for treatment of calcaneal fractures can be used to provide a flat, stable surface to support the operative limb distal to the operative site (Excel Medical Solutions, Plymouth MN) (**Fig. 5**).

Once the patient is positioned, special care attention needs to be made to protecting pressure areas, because the risk of pressure sores and neural injuries is higher in the obese patient.[31,33,34] The increased weight leads to increased pressure on contact points and makes it more difficult to properly position the unconscious obese patient safely. The table extensions and arm boards need to provide enough padding with sufficient size and strength to maintain proper positioning. Stretch injuries to the brachial plexus can occur during supine or prone positioning either from the arms being excessively abducted or from the weight of the patient's outstretched arm.[31,35] In the supine position, the arms need to be placed

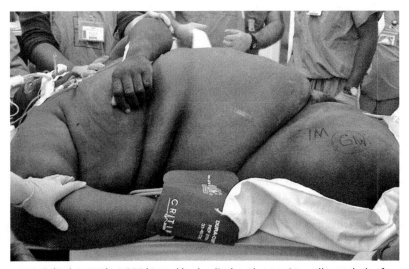

Fig. 4. This patient weighed more than 225 kg and had a displaced posterior wall acetabular fracture. Because of his girth, he required dual beanbags taped together to position him in the lateral position. (*Courtesy of* George V. Russell, MD.)

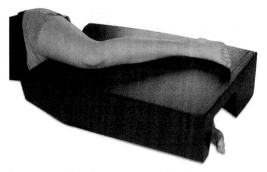

Fig. 5. A model demonstrating the leg tunnel. The author have found the leg tunnel useful when positioning patients in the lateral decubitus position for operative stabilization of acetabular fractures. The leg tunnel provides a stable platform to rest the operative leg, which is particularly helpful with obese and morbidly obese patients. (Excel Medical Solutions, Plymouth, MN) (*Courtesy of* George V. Russell, MD.)

on adequately padded arm boards to prevent the dorsal extension of the arm, which can stretch the plexus or put pressure on the ulnar nerve at the elbow. Perioperative ulnar neuropathy has been associated with increased body mass index (BMI, calculated as weight in kilograms divided by the square of height in meters).[36] Sciatic nerve palsies can occur from prolonged ischemic pressure associated with tilting the bed.[31] When placing the patient into the lateral decubitus position, care needs to be taken to protect the peroneal nerve on the nonoperative lower extremity.

The additional weight of the obese patient also makes them prone to pressure ulcers.[37] Pressure ulcers occur when the blood supply to the tissue is diminished, leading to ischemia, which can result in necrosis.[38] The main causes of pressure ulcers are pressure, shearing, and friction. Any external pressure greater than 32 mm Hg can cause capillary occlusion, limiting oxygen distally. The use of blankets and sheets can increase pressures by almost 44 mm Hg.[39] The increased mass from the obese patient creates more pressure because of their larger bodyweight loading on bony prominences, which in turn induces higher mechanical stress concentrations (ie, high forces per unit area of tissue) in their deep soft tissues (**Fig. 6**). There are reports of compartment syndromes attributed to poor positioning of the obese patient.[33,40] Surgical times as low as 2.5 to 4 hours have been shown to significantly increase the risk of postoperative pressure ulcer development.[41] Intraoperatively, patient warmers have been associated with the development of fewer pressure ulcers.[42] Avoiding hypotension and maintaining tissue perfusion and oxygenation further reduces the risk of pressure ulcer formation.

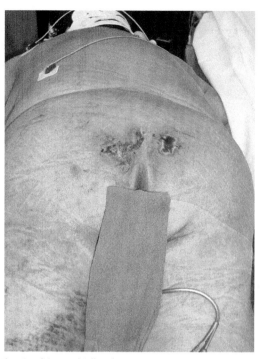

Fig. 6. This morbidly obese patient presented to the operating room 3 weeks after injury. Note the early pressure sores on the buttock. Despite the extra soft tissues creating a cushion, the increased patient weight promotes the formation of pressure sores. (*Courtesy of* George V. Russell, MD.)

Antibiotic Prophylaxis

The bioavailability of prophylactic antibiotics and anesthetic medications is affected by the increased amount of adipose tissue present in the obese patient. The physiologic changes related to obesity can change the volume of distribution, the amount of protein binding, the metabolism, and the elimination of drugs. The volume of distribution of lipophilic drugs is altered by the increased adipose tissue, and hydrophilic medications can be affected by the increased organ mass, decreased lean body mass, and increased blood volume and cardiac content.[43] These changes that occur with obesity can potentially lead to under- or overtherapeutic concentrations of medications. One study found in patients with a BMI greater than 50 kg/m^2 that 2 g of cefazolin only achieved therapeutic levels in 30% of tissues.[44] Aminoglycosides have been shown to require a dosing adjustment in obesity because of these altered pharmacokinetics; however, it has also been shown that simply dosing based on weight can lead to increase risk of toxicity.[43] To avoid overdosing in obesity, the change in the volume of distribution can be accounted for by a dosing weight correction factor.[43] Similarly, obese patients have been shown to have increased volumes of distribution and clearance of vancomycin through the kidneys, thus requiring level monitoring and weight-based dosing.[43] The available information for cephalosporins and other classes of antimicrobials suggests that dosages may need to be increased in obese compared with nonobese patients to attain similar effects.[45]

SURGICAL TIPS
General Considerations

Because anatomic reductions of the articular surface have been shown to lead to better results, open reduction and internal fixation is often mandated in patients with displaced acetabular fractures. The surgeon may need to modify standard techniques when operating on a pelvic or acetabular fracture in an obese patient. Surgical incisions must typically be extended to improve visualization of the bone. In addition, most instruments are poorly adapted for the large soft tissue envelope. Longer drills and deeper retractors are often required. The primary approaches to the acetabulum include the Kocher-Langenbeck and ilioinguinal approaches. The extended iliofemoral approach should probably be avoided given the higher rate of complications seen in nonobese patients and the extensive surgical dissection. For pelvic fractures, the Pfannensteil approach is most commonly used to access the anterior pelvis. Most surgeons use percutaneous fixation of the posterior pelvic ring. The ilioinguinal and Pfannensteil approaches may require incisions through the panniculus.

The distance between the soft tissue envelope and the underlying bone can result in difficulties identifying standard radiographic landmarks. These difficulties result in an increased dependence on fluoroscopy. However, as previously discussed for plain images and CT scans, intraoperative images may be difficult to obtain and interpret. The use of fluoroscopy may be altered because of the increased amount of subcutaneous adipose tissue. In addition, the typical aperture may not include the entire operative field in an obese patient. Increasing the kilovolts peak on the fluoroscopy machine can lead to improved penetration of adipose tissue.[10]

AUTHORS' PREFERRED PRACTICE: SURGICAL EXPOSURES
Anterior Surgical Exposures

The ilioinguinal, Pfannensteil and Stoppa exposures are commonly used in the operative treatment of acetabular fractures and pelvic ring injuries. Each of these exposures is more difficult in obese and morbidly obese patients. Exposure through the adipose layer to the deeper structures can be formidable. Sharp dissection is recommended through the adipose layer to decrease postoperative lipolysis and prolonged postoperative wound drainage. If possible, avoid incisions at the base of a pannicular fold. Incisions can frequently be moved proximal to the pannicular crease, incising through the panniculus itself (**Fig. 7**). Control of the adipose layer is usually achieved with self-retracting retractors and the aid of assistants using other retractors. One or two Charnley retractors may be required to provide adequate visualization, and even then it may prove impossible (**Fig. 8**).

Deep dissection and fracture exposure are difficult. Deep visualization is facilitated by extra-long skin incisions. A bump under the thigh will help to relieve tension on the iliopsoas muscle. Current retractors are often inappropriate to adequately retract to provide for optimal visualization. Additional assistants are frequently required to supplement current retractors. The authors use stiff malleable, Homan, Deever, Sofield retractors.

Pelvic exposure may be facilitated by using a modified Stoppa surgical exposure.[46] The modified Stoppa exposure, as described, provides visualization of the symphysis pubis, the anterior column of the acetabulum, the quadrilateral surface, the greater sciatic notch, and the sacroiliac joint. However, this extensive visualization is often compromised in obese patients. To improve visualization, a tenotomy of the rectus abdominis muscle may be performed just proximal to its insertion along the pelvic brim, providing improved access to the fracture and partially negating the effect of a large abdomen. At the termination of the procedure, the rectus tenotomy is repaired to both its insertion and the contralateral rectus abdominis muscle.

Posterior Exposures

The Kocher-Langenbeck surgical exposure is the most commonly used posterior approach for stabilizing acetabular fractures. The Kocher-Langenbeck exposure may be used in both the lateral and prone positions. The advantages of using the lateral position are easier patient positioning, easier ventilation, and surgeon familiarity. Using the lateral position, the posterior adipose sleeve falls back toward the surgeon, away from the surgical field. However, the trade-off is that one may be working at the bottom of a deep hole. Another potential disadvantage in using the

A

B

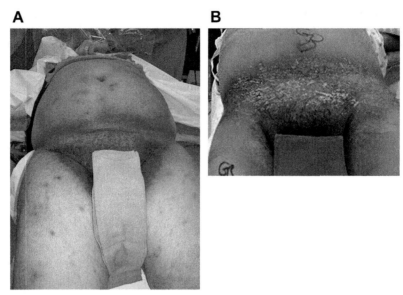

Fig. 7. (*A*) Preoperative view of proposed ilioinguinal surgical exposure site. Note the skin maceration and likely bacterial contamination. Consideration should be given to incising the skin through the panniculus to avoid this area. Also note the tinea cruris (jock itch) about the groin. (*B*) This patient had excessive skin flaking caused by poor hygiene. This flaking may increase the chances for postoperative infection. Although this patient is not extremely obese, a pannicular ring is noted in the valley of the overhanging panniculus. (*Courtesy of* George V. Russell, MD.)

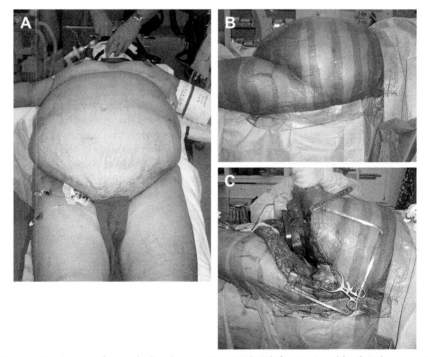

Fig. 8. (*A*) Preoperative image of a morbidly obese patient with a left associated both column acetabular fracture. (*B*) The surgical site has been sterilized and draped. The Ioban strips are noted about the surgical field. Ioban strips are preferred to Ioban sheets because of better contouring about the large abdomen and lower extremity. (*C*) Intraoperative images of retractors used to gain visualization during an ilioinguinal surgical exposure. A Charnley retractor was required. It is extremely difficult for the assistant to retract the large abdomen. (*Courtesy of* George V. Russell, MD.)

lateral position occurs with transverse fractures where the weight of the lower extremity will tend to displace the ischiopubic fracture segment medially.

Use of the Kocher-Langenbeck surgical exposure in the prone position has the advantage of less blood pooling in the depths of the wound and less medial displacement of fractures. However, there are many obstacles to overcome, and primary among them is retraction of the soft tissues as they fall into the operative field. Sharp dissection through the adipose layer is suggested to prevent postoperative lipolysis. A Charnley retractor is necessary for adequate visualization. Dual Charnley retractors may also be helpful for a large buttock. For the largest of buttocks, the Charnley retractor may need to be inset within the surgical incision because the blades are often not deep enough to retract the adipose tissues. Deep retraction is a problem, as it is for the anterior exposures with the exception of the use of extra-large sciatic nerve retractors (**Fig. 9**). Extra assistants are beneficial to retract the abundant soft tissues.

The vertical paramedian surgical exposure is required when open stabilization of posterior pelvic ring injuries is necessary. Historically, this exposure was associated with a high wound complication profile. Although this exposure is effective to allow access to the posterior pelvic ring for reductions of pelvic ring fractures and dislocations, the authors prefer not to use this exposure in patients who are morbidly obese. Attempts are made to stabilize posterior pelvic ring disruptions percutaneously in this patient population.

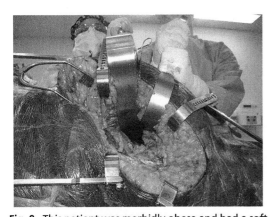

Fig. 9. This patient was morbidly obese and had a soft tissue envelope that measured 20 cm. Surgical visualization was difficult. Note an angled self-retaining retractor, 2 Charnley retractors, as well as 2 assistants on the opposite side of the table. The assistant on the left is using an extra-large sciatic nerve retractor. The assistant on the right is using a large Deaver retractor. (*Courtesy of* George V. Russell, MD.)

LITERATURE AND OUTCOMES

Patients who are obese have been shown to experience different injury patterns, with more thoracic, pelvic, and extremity injuries and fewer visceral or head injuries than patients who are not obese.[47] In addition, patients who are obese have been shown to have a 5 times higher mortality after trauma and an increased risk of infectious and noninfectious complications, including multiple organ failure, compared with patients who are not obese.[47,48] A recent study showed that obese patients experience a prolonged metabolic acidosis in severe blunt trauma that is associated with an increased incidence of multiple organ failure.[49] This is likely secondary to suboptimal resuscitation because standard trauma protocols are based on end points that inadequately account for the underlying metabolic abnormalities associated with obesity.

Concerns regarding surgical dissection through large amounts of soft tissue (and/or the panniculus) and risk of infection have led some surgeons to consider external fixation or limited techniques to avoid tissue injury in the treatment of pelvic fractures. Although the appeal of this technique is understandable, the practical application is difficult because the external fixator frequently impinges on the anterior abdominal soft tissues and is associated with a high rate of pin tract infections. Hupel and colleagues[50] reviewed their experience with external fixation in the treatment of rotationally unstable pelvic ring injuries and reported the consistent inability to maintain reduction compared with patients of normal weight.

Most of the current literature on the open treatment of pelvic and acetabular fractures in the obese has focused on complications. Pressure-related complications, including nerve palsies, and unusual complications such as thoracic level paraplegia have been reported.[51] However, most studies have focused on the increased risk of infection after the operative treatment of acetabular fractures. Karunakar and colleagues[5] identified a relationship with BMI and risk for complications, showing that incremental increases in BMI were associated with a higher risk of complications after open reduction and internal fixation of acetabular fractures. In this series, patients who were morbidly obese (BMI>40 kg/m^2) were 5 times more likely to have a wound infection than subjects of normal weight. Patients who were obese (BMI >30 kg/m^2) were 2.1 times more likely to have an estimated blood loss greater than 750 and 2.6 times more likely to develop a deep venous thrombosis (DVT). Porter and colleagues[3] corroborated these results in their series of patients who were morbidly obese (BMI>40 kg/m^2) and undergoing operative fixation of acetabular fractures. In this series, there was a 46% rate of wound complications compared with 12% in the nonmorbidly obese (BMI<40 kg/m^2). The overall rate of complications was 63% versus 24%, resulting in a relative increased risk of a 260% for the morbidly obese patients. Most complications were related to wound healing problems and were successfully controlled with aggressive surgical debridement (**Fig. 10**).

The same investigators also reported a complication rate for obese patients with operatively managed pelvic fractures twice that of the nonobese cohort.[4] Almost half of the reported complications were related to wound infections. They also noted a difference in injury pattern with a higher percentage of anteroposterior compression than lateral compression pelvic fractures. Sems and colleagues[6] reported a 54.2% complication rate after operative treatment of pelvic ring injuries in obese patients with a statistically higher rate of deep infection and loss of reduction greater than 1 cm in Tile type C fractures. They also noted

a correlation between BMI and increased rate of complications similar to that previously described for acetabular fractures.

The increased risk of infections in obese patients is likely multifactorial, with contributions from patient physiology (diabetes, perfusion), body habitus (subcutaneous tissue and panniculus and injury pattern), surgical time, and the trauma itself. The existence of a Morel Lavalee (internal degloving) lesion can also increase the risk of infection if not identified and managed aggressively with surgical debridement. Carlson and colleagues[52] identified an association between obesity and an increased risk of Morel Lavalee lesion requiring treatment. This association makes sense clinically because a larger layer of fat exposed to shear would have a higher risk of avulsion from the underlying fascia.

The high rate of infections and wound complications has also led to debate among surgeons concerning whether the indications and techniques for operative fixation of pelvic and acetabular fractures should be modified for the obese patient. The authors believe that attempts to reduce the

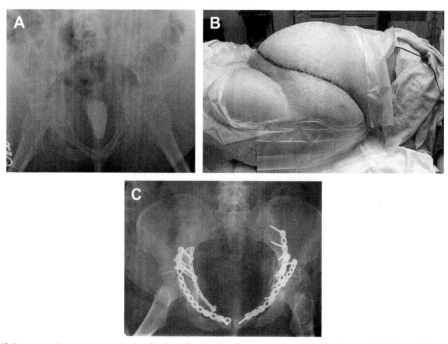

Fig. 10. (*A*) Preoperative anteroposterior (AP) radiograph of a morbidly obese patient with bilateral T-type acetabular fractures. Manual reduction efforts were attempted in the emergency room. Closed reduction was accomplished in the operating room. The patient required bilateral ilioinguinal surgical exposures as well as a left Kocher-Langenbeck exposure for operative fracture reduction and stabilization. This patient also underwent a rectus abdominis tenotomy on the right side to improve operative visualization and implant placement. (*B*) Intraoperative clinical image of patient during a subsequent debridement and irrigation procedure. This patient underwent 12 operative debridements to control postoperative wound drainage. (*C*) Postoperative AP pelvic radiograph 11 months after open reduction and fixation of her acetabular fractures. (*Courtesy of* George V. Russell, MD.)

risk of infection should be made, but that indications should not change simply for obesity. Further details on the topic of minimally invasive pelvic and acetabular surgery are covered elsewhere in this issue.

There are currently no published data on the longer-term follow-up or functional outcomes of operatively treated pelvic and acetabular fractures in the obese patient. Many clinicians question the ability to achieve anatomic or near-anatomic fracture reductions in this challenging patient population. Research is currently ongoing to evaluate these issues. However, the authors believe, based on their clinical experience, that the functional outcomes are similar to those of patients who are not obese if an anatomic reduction can be obtained, and complications, when present, are addressed early and aggressively.

UNDERSTANDING AND PREVENTING COMPLICATIONS
Wound Infections

Surgical site infections (SSI) occur with increased frequency in trauma patients who are obese and are associated with significant perioperative morbidity.[3,5,37,48] This increased risk is likely multifactorial, with components attributable to local tissue characteristics (see **Fig. 7**), surgical trauma, and patient physiology. Adipose tissue is poorly vascularized, resulting in suboptimal tissue perfusion and insufficient oxygenation that can lead to compromised wound healing through effects on collagen synthesis, angiogenesis, and epithelialization.[53,54] The larger surface area required for surgical exposure in the obese patient further exacerbates the effects of poor vascularization. The increased adipose tissue can put more pressure on the wound edges, decreasing blood flow to the tissues and increasing the risk of wound dehiscence.[55] In addition, the presence of excess fat can prolong operative time, and require longer and more forceful retraction, resulting in more tissue trauma, leading to increased rates of infections.[56,57]

Obesity is a surrogate for other known risk factors associated with SSI. There is a strong correlation between obesity and the development of type II diabetes. Postoperative hyperglycemia has been shown to be associated with surgical infections in patients with and without diabetes.[12,24,25,58] Operative procedures in the obese are associated with increased blood loss, higher transfusion requirements and increased operative times, all of which are associated with increased risk of infection.[3–6] Obesity itself is an intrinsic risk factor that has systemic effects that alter the cardiovascular, respiratory, and inflammatory or healing processes, creating conditions that increase the risk of SSI.

In the obese patient, the workload of the heart is frequently increased by the strain of supplying blood to all tissues. Normal wound healing depends on the circulatory system to provide oxygen and nutrients. Ischemia, or a lack of blood to the tissue, can lead to necrosis. Because adipose tissue is already poorly vascularized, it is less tolerant of ischemia and hypoxemia than the epidermis.[59] Obese patients typically present with a hypoventilation respiratory pattern resulting from the inability of the diaphragm to fully descend because of abdominal adipose tissue. Chest expansion is impaired, resulting in decreased vital capacity and tidal function, which compromises tissue oxygenation and may adversely affect wound healing. Basic science studies have suggested that fibroblasts need an oxygen pressure greater than 15 mm Hg for adequate collagen formation.[54]

Given the well-documented risk of SSI infection in the obese patient the surgeon should attempt to minimize all controllable risk factors. Procedure-related risk factors include poor surgical technique, duration of the surgery, quality of skin preparation, and inadequate sterilization of surgical instruments.[60] Good surgical technique requires obtaining hemostasis, removal of all devitalized tissue, and elimination of dead space at the surgical site.[61] Preoperatively, appropriate weight-based doses of prophylactic antibiotics administered within 30 minutes of incision and a thorough preparation of all soft tissue folds with an alcohol-based surgical preparatory solution should be performed. Strict perioperative control of hyperglycemia with an insulin drip, or at least an adjusted basal bolus dosing regimen, should be considered. Supplemental administration of oxygen with an increased perioperative forced inspiratory oxygen (Fio^2), to maximize incisional oxygen tension, may also help to increase tissue oxygenation during longer procedures.[62] Surgical techniques for wound closure and tissue handling include atraumatic tissue handling, debridement of devitalized tissue, continuous fascial closure, closure of subcutaneous fat, and optimizing suture length/wound length ratio.[37] There has been a recent enthusiasm for negative pressure therapy with incisional wound vacuum-assisted closure (VAC) placement. Reddix and colleagues[63] reported on the successful use of incisional VAC in reducing wound complications in a series of 19 morbidly obese patients.

Postoperatively soiled bandages should be changed frequently and hematoma or seromas should be aggressively managed. In general, persistent wound drainage after 7 days rarely stops, and requires surgical debridement and repeat closure. If the surgeon is concerned about the presence of a hematoma or seroma, a CT scan or ultrasound can be considered to evaluate for a fluid collection.

Many obese patients are not well nourished. In order for wounds to heal, the body needs a positive nitrogen balance (defined as the difference between nitrogen intake and excretion). Serum albumin is the major protein synthesized by the liver and plays a role in maintaining plasma oncotic pressure, delivery of metabolites, enzymes, drugs, and hormones in the blood stream, and facilitates wound healing. During trauma, albumin synthesis decreases and albumin use increases at wound sites. A low serum albumin is an indicator of impaired wound healing. Simple interventions such as dietary supplements (to increase protein) will help create a positive nitrogen balance and may improve wound healing.

AUTHORS' PREFERRED PRACTICE: PREVENTION OF WOUND INFECTIONS

The authors recommend the use of sharp dissection with a scalpel through the subcutaneous adipose tissue layer and avoiding electrocautery dissection to minimize further devascularization of the fatty tissue. On completion of the procedure, all devitalized adipose tissue should be sharply debrided. Multiple suture layers in the subcutaneous layers reduce tissue sheer and decrease potential dead space, which may help to reduce wound complications. Drains should be used when significant bleeding or dead space remain. The authors have used the incisional wound VAC with initial positive results. The wound VAC addresses 2 principle problems encountered in morbidly obese patients. First, lipolysis and prolonged drainage frequently occur. As the fat drains from the wound, a pathway is created whereby bacteria may gain entrance within the wound. Second, because the patients are large and often perspire about their incision, it is difficult to achieve a tape seal about the wound, which then potentiates the first problem. The incisional wound VAC addresses both of these problems by creating a sterile environment that may be maintained for several days. Our protocol at the completion of surgery is to place incisional wound VACs on morbidly obese patients. The wound is checked no sooner than 72 hours after surgery. If the wound is dry, then standard dry dressing changes are initiated. If the wound is not dry, we reapply the wound VAC for another 48 to 72 hours. Another inspection is then performed. If the wound is dry, no further treatment is needed. If the wound continues to drain, then an irrigation and debridement is performed.

DVT AND PULMONARY EMBOLISM

Obesity is an independent risk factor for DVT and pulmonary embolism (PE).[29,64] Major orthopedic trauma patients have a risk of 10% to 30% of having a proximal DVT, 1.3% to 10% of clinically relevant PE, and 0.2% to 5% of a fatal PE.[65,66] Obese trauma patients are also likely at an increased risk because of further limitations in their mobility related to surgery and associated injuries. Karunakar and colleagues[5] showed a 2.6 times higher rate of DVT in obese patients compared with nonobese patients. The relationship between DVT and obesity stems from the increased intra-abdominal pressure and venous stasis associated with central obesity, which creates a hypercoagulable state.[32] These effects are accentuated by anesthesia-induced paralysis and postoperative limitations in motion. From a cellular stand point, obese patients have increased fasting plasma fatty acid levels, which accelerate the coagulation cascade.[48] Obesity has also been shown to create a hypercoagulable state with increased levels of fibrinogen, factor VIII, and von Willebrand factor. In addition, obesity is associated with a decrease in fibrinolytic activity.[48] The duration of a pelvic or acetabular surgery is frequently prolonged, further amplifying this risk.

Screening and diagnosing a DVT or PE can be more difficult in the obese patient. The detection of swelling in the limbs of an obese patient can be harder to appreciate on physical examination. Venous Doppler ultrasound of legs is one of the main screening tools for the diagnosis of a DVT. This test can be less diagnostic in the obese patient because the ultrasound beams can be attenuated by the increased fat, limiting image quality.[10] Evaluation for PE is typically performed with a CT scan and suffers similar limitations, as previously discussed.

Postoperatively, some form of prophylaxis is recommended for the prevention of a venous thromboembolic event. The mechanical methods of prophylaxis, intermittent pneumatic leg compression and graduated compression stockings, can be difficult to use in the obese and have not been adequately studied for effectiveness in this population. Oral anticoagulants or low molecular weight heparins (LMWH) are the preferred pharmacologic methods. When considering their use, the side effect of bleeding requires further consideration because the obese patient is more prone to wound complications.[67] There is controversy about whether the obese patient requires larger doses of anticoagulants to obtain therapeutic levels.[65] The LMWH have been shown to have decreased subcutaneous absorption and increased volume of distribution in the obese patient.[45] One study showed benefit from the use of a higher fixed dose of LMWH.[68] Further research is needed to fully determine the dosing in obese patients; however, increasing doses and longer duration should be considered.[69]

HETEROTOPIC OSSIFICATION

Heterotopic ossification is a well-known complication of operative management of acetabular fractures, associated most strongly with the Kocher-Langenbeck approach. The use of a prophylactic regimen with either indomethacin or radiation is controversial, with no clear consensus existing in the literature. A recent meta-analysis supports the superiority of low-dose irradiation compared with indomethacin.[70] Both Karunakar and colleagues[5] and Porter and colleagues[3] were unable to show a relationship between obesity and heterotopic ossification. The decision on the method and indications for prophylaxis should be made by the treating surgeon on an individual patient basis.

LOSS OF FIXATION, MALUNION, ARTHRITIS

There are currently limited data on the incidence of loss of fixation, malunion, and development of arthritis for the obese patient with an operatively treated pelvic or acetabular fracture. Porter and colleagues[4] reported a 10% rate of implant or fixation failure compared with 1% in the nonobese group in their series of pelvic fracture patients. Sems and colleagues[6] reported a 31% rate of fixation failure after internal fixation of pelvic fractures for obese patients compared with a 6% rate for nonobese patients. For acetabular fractures, the development of arthritis has been most commonly associated with the quality of reduction. Although there are no specific studies, it is likely that this association also holds true for obese patients.

SUMMARY

The open operative management of pelvic and acetabular fractures in the obese is technically demanding, with a significantly higher rate of complications compared with patients who are not obese. The decision to perform surgery should involve a thorough understanding of risks, and patients should be counseled. Careful attention should be paid to patient factors; coexisting systemic conditions and patient positioning can reduce complications. Wound complications are most commonly seen, and techniques to reduce risk should be incorporated. When complications occur, aggressive management can result in successful salvage. Future areas of study should include methods to reduce risk of SSI and improving understanding of the physiologic alterations that occur with obesity.

REFERENCES

1. Kopelman PG. Obesity as a medical problem. Nature 2000;404:635–43.
2. Mokdad AH, Ford ES, Bowman BA, et al. Prevalence of obesity, diabetes, and obesity-related health risk factors, 2001. JAMA 2003;289:76–9.
3. Porter SE, Russell GV, Dews RC, et al. Complications of acetabular fracture surgery in morbidly obese patients. J Orthop Trauma 2008;22:589–94.
4. Porter SE, Graves ML, Qin Z, et al. Operative experience of pelvic fractures in the obese. Obes Surg 2008;18:702–8.
5. Karunakar MA, Shah SN, Jerabek S. Body mass index as a predictor of complications after operative treatment of acetabular fractures. J Bone Joint Surg Am 2005;87:1498–502.
6. Sems SA, Johnson M, Cole PA, et al. Elevated body mass index increases early complications of surgical treatment of pelvic ring injuries. J Orthop Trauma 2010;24:309–14.
7. Bullo M, Casas-Agustench P, Amigo-Correig P, et al. Inflammation, obesity and comorbidities: the role of diet. Public Health Nutr 2007;10:1164–72.
8. Must A, Spadano J, Coakley EH, et al. The disease burden associated with overweight and obesity. JAMA 1999;282:1523–9.
9. Brunette DD. Resuscitation of the morbidly obese patient. Am J Emerg Med 2004;22:40–7.
10. Uppot RN. Impact of obesity on radiology. Radiol Clin North Am 2007;45:231–46.
11. Ginde AA, Foianini A, Renner DM, et al. The challenge of CT and MRI imaging of obese individuals who present to the emergency department: a national survey. Obesity (Silver Spring) 2008;16:2549–51.
12. Wellen KE, Hotamisligil GS. Inflammation, stress, and diabetes. J Clin Invest 2005;115:1111–9.
13. Hossain P, Kawar B, El NM. Obesity and diabetes in the developing world—a growing challenge. N Engl J Med 2007;356:213–5.
14. Wild S, Roglic G, Green A, et al. Global prevalence of diabetes: estimates for the year 2000 and projections for 2030. Diabetes Care 2004;27:1047–53.
15. Demaria EJ, Carmody BJ. Perioperative management of special populations: obesity. Surg Clin North Am 2005;85:1283–9, xii.

16. Shenkman Z, Shir Y, Brodsky JB. Perioperative management of the obese patient. Br J Anaesth 1993;70:349–59.

17. Belzberg H, Wo CC, Demetriades D, et al. Effects of age and obesity on hemodynamics, tissue oxygenation, and outcome after trauma. J Trauma 2007;62:1192–200.

18. Ray CS, Sue DY, Bray G, et al. Effects of obesity on respiratory function. Am Rev Respir Dis 1983;128:501–6.

19. Biring MS, Lewis MI, Liu JT, et al. Pulmonary physiologic changes of morbid obesity. Am J Med Sci 1999;318:293–7.

20. Flancbaum L, Choban PS. Surgical implications of obesity. Annu Rev Med 1998;49:215–34.

21. Martyn JA, Kaneki M, Yasuhara S. Obesity-induced insulin resistance and hyperglycemia: etiologic factors and molecular mechanisms. Anesthesiology 2008;109:137–48.

22. Saltiel AR, Kahn CR. Insulin signalling and the regulation of glucose and lipid metabolism. Nature 2001;414:799–806.

23. Hansen TK, Thiel S, Wouters PJ, et al. Intensive insulin therapy exerts antiinflammatory effects in critically ill patients and counteracts the adverse effect of low mannose-binding lectin levels. J Clin Endocrinol Metab 2003;88:1082–8.

24. Turina M, Fry DE, Polk HC Jr. Acute hyperglycemia and the innate immune system: clinical, cellular, and molecular aspects. Crit Care Med 2005;33:1624–33.

25. Digman C, Borto D, Nasraway SA Jr. Hyperglycemia in the critically ill. Nutr Clin Care 2005;8:93–101.

26. Geerlings SE, Hoepelman AI. Immune dysfunction in patients with diabetes mellitus (DM). FEMS Immunol Med Microbiol 1999;26:259–65.

27. Carr JM, Sellke FW, Fey M, et al. Implementing tight glucose control after coronary artery bypass surgery. Ann Thorac Surg 2005;80:902–9.

28. Czupryniak L, Strzelczyk J, Pawlowski M, et al. Mild elevation of fasting plasma glucose is a strong risk factor for postoperative complications in gastric bypass patients. Obes Surg 2004;14:1393–7.

29. Abir F, Bell R. Assessment and management of the obese patient. Crit Care Med 2004;32:S87–91.

30. Hunt D. Evaluating equipment and techniques for safe perioperative positioning of the morbidly obese patient. Bariatric Nursing and Surgical Patient Care 2007;2:57–63.

31. Ogunnaike BO, Jones SB, Jones DB, et al. Anesthetic considerations for bariatric surgery. Anesth Analg 2002;95:1793–805.

32. Adams JP, Murphy PG. Obesity in anaesthesia and intensive care. Br J Anaesth 2000;85:91–108.

33. Jupiter JB, Ring D, Rosen H. The complications and difficulties of management of nonunion in the severely obese. J Orthop Trauma 1995;9:363–70.

34. Bamgbade OA, Rutter TW, Nafiu OO, et al. Postoperative complications in obese and nonobese patients. World J Surg 2007;31:556–60.

35. Winfree CJ, Kline DG. Intraoperative positioning nerve injuries. Surg Neurol 2005;63:5–18.

36. Warner MA, Warner ME, Martin JT. Ulnar neuropathy. Incidence, outcome, and risk factors in sedated or anesthetized patients. Anesthesiology 1994;81:1332–40.

37. Derzie AJ, Silvestri F, Liriano E, et al. Wound closure technique and acute wound complications in gastric surgery for morbid obesity: a prospective randomized trial. J Am Coll Surg 2000;191:238–43.

38. Pokorny ME. Skin physiology and diseases in the obese patient. Bariatric Nursing and Surgical Patient Care 2008;3:125–8.

39. Schultz A, Bien M, Dumond K, et al. Etiology and incidence of pressure ulcers in surgical patients. AORN J 1999;70:434–49.

40. Wiltshire JP, Custer T. Lumbar muscle rhabdomyolysis as a cause of acute renal failure after Roux-en-Y gastric bypass. Obes Surg 2003;13:306–13.

41. Aronovitch SA. Intraoperatively acquired pressure ulcer prevalence: a national study. Adv Wound Care 1998;11:8–9.

42. Scott EM, Leaper DJ, Clark M, et al. Effects of warming therapy on pressure ulcers—a randomized trial. AORN J 2001;73:921–33, 936.

43. Bearden DT, Rodvold KA. Dosage adjustments for antibacterials in obese patients: applying clinical pharmacokinetics. Clin Pharmacokinet 2000;38:415–26.

44. Edmiston CE, Krepel C, Kelly H, et al. Perioperative antibiotic prophylaxis in the gastric bypass patient: do we achieve therapeutic levels? Surgery 2004;136:738–47.

45. Lee JB, Winstead PS, Cook AM. Pharmacokinetic alterations in obesity. Orthopedics 2006;29:984–8.

46. Cole JD, Bolhofner BR. Acetabular fracture fixation via a modified Stoppa limited intrapelvic approach. Description of operative technique and preliminary treatment results. Clin Orthop Relat Res 1994;305:112–23.

47. Boulanger BR, Milzman D, Mitchell K, et al. Body habitus as a predictor of injury pattern after blunt trauma. J Trauma 1992;33:228–32.

48. Choban PS, Flancbaum L. The impact of obesity on surgical outcomes: a review. J Am Coll Surg 1997;185:593–603.

49. Winfield RD, Delano MJ, Lottenberg L, et al. Traditional resuscitative practices fail to resolve metabolic acidosis in morbidly obese patients after severe blunt trauma. J Trauma 2010;68:317–30.

50. Hupel TM, McKee MD, Waddell JP, et al. Primary external fixation of rotationally unstable pelvic fractures in obese patients. J Trauma 1998;45:111–5.

51. Russell GV Jr, Nork SE, Chip RM Jr. Perioperative complications associated with operative treatment

of acetabular fractures. J Trauma 2001;51: 1098–103.

52. Carlson DA, Simmons J, Sando W, et al. Morel-Lavalee lesions treated with debridement and meticulous dead space closure: surgical technique. J Orthop Trauma 2007;21:140–4.

53. Rosell S, Belfrage E. Blood circulation in adipose tissue. Physiol Rev 1979;59:1078–104.

54. Wilson JA, Clark JJ. Obesity: impediment to postsurgical wound healing. Adv Skin Wound Care 2004;17: 426–35.

55. Armstrong D, Bortz P. An integrative review of pressure relief in surgical patients. AORN J 2001;73: 645–53, 656.

56. Gong EM, Orvieto MA, Lyon MB, et al. Analysis of impact of body mass index on outcomes of laparoscopic renal surgery. Urology 2007;69:38–43.

57. Canturk Z, Canturk NZ, Cetinarslan B, et al. Nosocomial infections and obesity in surgical patients. Obes Res 2003;11:769–75.

58. Goldberg PA, Sakharova OV, Barrett PW, et al. Improving glycemic control in the cardiothoracic intensive care unit: clinical experience in two hospital settings. J Cardiothorac Vasc Anesth 2004;18:690–7.

59. Chesser TJS, Hammettt RB, Norton SA. Orthopaedic trauma in the obese patient. Injury 2010;41:247–52.

60. Mangram AJ, Horan TC, Pearson ML, et al. Guideline for prevention of surgical site infection, 1999. Centers for Disease Control and Prevention (CDC) Hospital Infection Control Practices Advisory Committee. Am J Infect Control 1999;27:97–132.

61. Owens CD, Stoessel K. Surgical site infections: epidemiology, microbiology and prevention. J Hosp Infect 2008;70(Suppl 2):3–10.

62. Qadan M, Akca O, Mahid SS, et al. Perioperative supplemental oxygen therapy and surgical site infection: a meta-analysis of randomized controlled trials. Arch Surg 2009;144:359–66.

63. Reddix RN Jr, Tyler HK, Kulp B, et al. Incisional vacuum-assisted wound closure in morbidly obese patients undergoing acetabular fracture surgery. Am J Orthop (Belle Mead NJ) 2009;38: 446–9.

64. Blaszyk H, Bjornsson J. Factor V Leiden and morbid obesity in fatal postoperative pulmonary embolism. Arch Surg 2000;135:1410–3.

65. Geerts WH, Bergqvist D, Pineo GF, et al. Prevention of venous thromboembolism: American College of Chest Physicians Evidence-Based Clinical Practice Guidelines (8th edition). Chest 2008;133:381S–453S.

66. Slavik RS, Chan E, Gorman SK, et al. Dalteparin versus enoxaparin for venous thromboembolism prophylaxis in acute spinal cord injury and major orthopedic trauma patients: 'DETECT' trial. J Trauma 2007;62:1075–81.

67. Choban PS, Heckler R, Burge JC, et al. Increased incidence of nosocomial infections in obese surgical patients. Am Surg 1995;61:1001–5.

68. Hamad GG, Choban PS. Enoxaparin for thromboprophylaxis in morbidly obese patients undergoing bariatric surgery: findings of the prophylaxis against VTE outcomes in bariatric surgery patients receiving enoxaparin (PROBE) study. Obes Surg 2005;15: 1368–74.

69. Nutescu EA, Spinler SA, Wittkowsky A, et al. Low-molecular-weight heparins in renal impairment and obesity: available evidence and clinical practice recommendations across medical and surgical settings. Ann Pharmacother 2009;43:1064–83.

70. Blokhuis TJ, Frolke JP. Is radiation superior to indomethacin to prevent heterotopic ossification in acetabular fractures?: a systematic review. Clin Orthop Relat Res 2009;467:526–30.

Evaluation and Treatment of Spinal Injuries in the Obese Patient

Robert M. Greenleaf, MD[a,b], Daniel T. Altman, MD[c],*

KEYWORDS

- Obese • Obesity • Spine • Injury • Trauma

Given the increasing incidence and severity of obesity in the adult population,[1] orthopaedic surgeons are evaluating and treating more acutely injured obese patients. Management of obese patients with spinal injuries and disorders is complicated given their body habitus and associated medical comorbidities. Although evaluation and treatment are almost the same as for nonobese patients, some special considerations are necessary to prevent errors in diagnosis and treatment of obese trauma patients. Predisposition to spinal injury, effective evaluation and early management, principles of treatment planning, operative technical pearls, and postoperative management are discussed.

PREDISPOSITION TO SPINAL INJURY

Studies on the relationship between obesity and spinal disease have focused primarily on degenerative changes and low back pain.[2–11] Much less is understood about the relationship between obesity and spinal injury. A large body habitus can make gross inspection and palpation of an injury difficult, placing greater importance on clinical suspicion and imaging. Determining if obesity predisposes blunt trauma patients to spinal injury could help guide evaluation in the emergency setting.

Data on the relationship between obesity and spinal injury after blunt trauma are sparse. Obesity is highly correlated with sleep apnea.[12,13] Sleep apnea leads to a 7-fold risk for motor vehicle accidents.[14,15] Brown and colleagues[16] performed a retrospective review of 1153 blunt trauma patients requiring admission to the intensive care unit comparing obese (body mass index [BMI], calculated as weight in kilograms divided by the square of height in meters >30 kg/m^2) and nonobese patients. Obese patients had significantly fewer head injuries but more chest and lower extremity injuries. There was no difference in the overall incidence of spinal fractures (14% vs 16% in obese vs nonobese) or the anatomic region involved. Bolaunger and colleagues[17] prospectively evaluated 743 obese blunt trauma patients. Obese patients had a higher incidence of rib fractures, pulmonary contusions, pelvic fractures, and extremity fractures, and were less likely to have incurred head trauma and liver injuries. Again, no significant relationship between obesity and spinal injury or type of injury was found.

INITIAL EVALUATION AND EARLY MANAGEMENT

The principles of acute trauma care are no different in obese patients versus nonobese patients. Following the ABCs and complete

Daniel T. Altman received Institutional support from Synthes; Robert M. Greenleaf - nothing to disclose.
a Allegheny General Hospital, Pittsburgh, PA, USA
b 1 Emerson Place Apartment, 12 North, Boston, MA 02114, USA
c Department of Orthopaedic Surgery, Allegheny General Hospital, Drexel University College of Medicine, Pittsburgh, PA, USA
* Corresponding author. 1307 Federal Street, 2nd floor, Pittsburgh, PA 15212.
E-mail address: Daltman@wpahs.org

Orthop Clin N Am 42 (2011) 85–93
doi:10.1016/j.ocl.2010.08.007
0030-5898/11/$ – see front matter © 2011 Elsevier Inc. All rights reserved.

removal of clothing and exposure, care should be directed toward a meticulous clinical evaluation. Spinal immobilization may be more difficult in the obese patient given heavier extremities, a relatively short, thick neck region, poorly fitting cervical collars, or problems fitting and transporting patients on the gurney. Sandbags may help augment cervical stabilization, or 1 person may need to be dedicated to holding in-line cervical traction if there is suspicion for cervical injury. To maintain spinal precautions during a log roll, additional personnel are needed and palpation of the spine should be deeper and more focused.

Imaging

Thorough imaging is paramount in any obese blunt trauma patient. Plain radiographs in obese patients may be of poor quality for several reasons. The large soft tissue envelope makes obtaining accurate images of the correct anatomy difficult for inexperienced technician. Also, the amount of penetration necessary may deteriorate the quality of the image. Body habitus and difficulty depressing the shoulders makes inclusion of the cervicothoracic junction on lateral cervical radiographs nearly impossible. Magnification error may be an issue. Ravi and Rampersaud[18] showed that linear clinical measurements obtained on digital radiographs are subject to significant magnification errors based on the patient's BMI. Consequently, clinical decision making that is based on linear measurements obtained from radiographs that do not account for this error is invalid. They suggest that in a scenario where this measurement is crucial, such as during dynamic radiographs or measuring for signs of instability in the cervical spine, this error can be corrected by comparison with morphometric data from computed tomography (CT) or magnetic resonance imaging (MRI).[19]

CT provides rapid, accurate bony images and has largely supplanted plain radiography for the evaluation of spinal injury. The Eastern Association for the Surgery of Trauma (EAST; http://www.east.org/tpg.asp)[19] recommended in its 2009 update, using CT as the only screening modality as plain radiographs do not contribute any additional information. However, a potential problem may arise with size limitations of the CT scanner. Ginde and colleagues[20] performed a detailed survey of 262 nonacademic and 136 academic hospitals across the United States to determine the characteristics of available CT scanners. In the nonacademic hospitals, 25% of CT scanners had a maximum weight limit of 159 kg (350 pounds) and only 10% could accommodate patients

more than 204 kg (450 pounds). At academic hospitals, 10% had limits of 159 kg and 21% could scan patients more than 204 kg. Only 21% of centers designated as Bariatric Centers of Excellence had large-weight CT capacity equipment. To determine if a large animal scanner is available to image heavier patients, the investigators also surveyed 145 zoos and veterinary hospitals. Only 2 zoos had large animal scanners but both refused to allow human imaging. Sixteen veterinary hospitals had large scanners (up to 907 kg [2000 pounds]) but 12 of these had strict policies prohibiting human use. If faced with this dilemma, the morbidly obese patient may need to be transported long distances to a facility with appropriate imaging capabilities.[20]

The obese patient may also be difficult to image with MRI. In evaluating MRI capabilities, 64% of nonacademic and 59% of academic facilities had a weight limit of 159 kg for their MRI scanners. Weight limits of 159 kg or a body diameter of 60 cm are common and prohibitive for effective MRI imaging in obese patients. Open-system MRI scanners can accommodate significantly larger patients but the images are often poor quality. Other difficulties include increased transport time, positioning, and longer scan time, which leads to patient discomfort and motion with resulting poor quality images.[20]

Early Medical Management

The medical comorbidities associated with obesity and the subsequent perioperative medical management were discussed in a previous article. Optimization of pulmonary function and toilet, oxygenation, blood counts, venous thromboembolism prophylaxis, and nutritional assessment are vital for successful outcomes.

TREATMENT PLANNING

Classification systems and treatment algorithms guiding spinal injury treatment are constantly evolving. The Spine Trauma Study Group has proposed more comprehensive classification systems for both cervical and thoracolumbar injury, helping to guide operative versus nonoperative treatment. These systems improve on previous systems by factoring in 3 important parameters: injury morphology, neurologic status, and integrity of soft tissue supports including posterior ligaments and intervertebral discs.[21,22] Body habitus is another important patient characteristic that should be considered when determining operative versus nonoperative treatment as nonoperative stabilization of a spinal injury in an obese patient may not be feasible with the commonly used rigid orthoses.

Bracing

The absolute surgical indications for patients with spinal injuries are (1) progressive neurologic deficit in the presence of surgically correctable compression or (2) instability or unstable ligamentous injury. Nonoperative care and/or bracing are valid options in most other injuries. However, bracing should be approached as a complex treatment option requiring close monitoring for signs of failure or complications. A large body habitus impairs 3- or 4-point immobilization necessary for orthotic immobilization at all spinal levels. Thus, motion at the involved spinal levels still occurs despite proper fitting. Evidence of bracing failure in obese patients is most evident in scoliosis treatment.[23,24] In the obese patient, the brace offers less mechanical support of the spine and is frequently not as well tolerated compared with thinner patients.[24] Given the inefficiency and complications from bracing and the large lever arm placed on the spine by a large ventral panniculus, the authors believe that strong consideration should be given to surgical fixation of potentially unstable thoracolumbar injuries in obese patients.

OPERATIVE PEARLS AND PITFALLS
Surgical Exposure

The surgical exposure should be dictated by the involved pathologic anatomy as in nonobese patients. Dorsal approaches and the anterior cervical Smith-Robinson approach are more difficult in obese patients and may require technique and equipment modifications as discussed later. Ventral approaches to the thoracolumbar spine are significantly deeper given the large panniculus. Complications from this approach were prospectively studied by Peng and colleagues[11] in 74 cases of obese versus nonobese patients for degenerative pathology. Although obese patients did require longer surgical duration and a larger incision, there were no significant differences in blood loss, analgesic use, time to ambulation or discharge, and complications. All of their cases were performed by a single experienced vascular access surgeon at a major academic center. Such an experienced access surgeon should be available for this approach.

Operating Table

The Amsco surgical table (Amsco 3085, Steris Corp, Montgomery, AL, USA) is our basic mobile surgical table and can accommodate 454 kg (1000 pounds) in its normal orientation. To facilitate intraoperative imaging, the head section can be inserted into the leg section. This orientation can only hold 227 kg (500 pounds). If the patient is too wide, 2 tables may be placed side-by-side in opposite orientations. Adapters for 3-point cranial fixation or traction tongs can be attached to the top of the bed.

Allowing the abdomen to hang free in the prone position facilitates vena cava decompression, decreased venous pressure in the operative field, and less operative blood loss. The spinal Jackson table (Mizuho OSI, Union City, CA, USA) allows this, is radiolucent, and can hold up to 227 kg. The table delivers automatic massage to its pads and pressure points and can be rotated for 360-degree fusion without repositioning the patient.

Positioning

Patient positioning should allow optimal exposure and visualization of the spinal segment involved while ensuring patient safety. Anesthesia concerns were discussed in a previous article and are of paramount concern. Patient positioning should safely place the anatomy in an optimal position for the desired procedure, that is, cervical extension or lumbar flexion for decompression or flexion/extension for reduction of traumatic deformities. There should be access for obtaining localizing radiographs. In a 2004 review, Goodkin and Laska[25] found that "(a) large body habitus or operating table limitations preventing adequate radiographic visualization of the operative level" was one of the most common causes of wrong level surgery.

Specific Positions
Supine position
The supine position permits exposure of the anterior spine via an anterior cervical, transthoracic, or transabdominal approach. The anterior cervical approach may be complicated by excessive tissue around the neck and submandibular panniculus. Cervical extension as tolerated helps to smooth out skin folds. Chin straps or tape with a topical adhesive may be used. Tape is placed from the lateral shoulder to the base of the bed to depress the shoulder for lateral cervical radiographs. However, care should be taken not to place excess traction. Roh and colleagues[26] evaluated the usefulness of somatosensory evoked potential monitoring during 809 consecutive cervical spine surgeries. In 2.1% of cases, positioning led to a critical change in somatosensory evoked potentials. The most common corrective maneuver was

release of tape and traction. Arm boards may be attached to the side of the bed and a sheet can be wrapped around the body and secured with tape for arm support.

Prone positioning

Compared with other positions, the prone position has the greatest potential for respiratory compromise manifested by increased peak airway pressure and abdominal compression manifested by increased venous congestion.[27] The spinal Jackson table best minimizes these problems. This table also has customized padding to minimize compression at pressure points. The head should be placed in stable foam padding in a neutral position. The arms should not be hyperabducted or extended over the head to protect from peripheral nerve or brachial plexus traction injury. The axillae should be free or padded without compression. The transverse chest support should be at the nipple line, the cephalad hip support is on the anterior superior iliac spine, and the caudal support at the mid to proximal thigh. The abdominal panniculus, genitalia, and Foley catheter should hang freely. Reston or an equivalent padding is placed under the knees and blankets are placed under the feet to affect at least 20 degrees of flexion at the knee. Make sure that

no body part is resting directly on any lines, tubes, cords, drains, or compression devices (**Fig. 1**).

Operative Complications

Data on perioperative complications in obese patients has come from reviews of elective surgeries for degenerative spinal conditions. Yadla and colleagues[2] prospectively studied the perioperative complications in 87 consecutive elective degenerative thoracolumbar procedures. The investigators concluded that BMI did not correlate with the incidence of minor, major, or any complications. However, several studies using similar methods reported an increase in complications. Patel and colleagues[9] retrospectively reviewed 86 surgeries for degenerative thoracolumbar disease. The investigators of this study correlated increasing BMI with increasing risk of major perioperative complications but not minor complications. These risks were also associated with increased age and increased number of levels. The investigators also noted that peripheral nerve palsies occurred only in the morbidly obese patients (BMI >40 kg/m^2). Peripheral nerve palsies are a known complication of the prone position in obese patients.[9] Preventative measures include meticulous padding of pressure points with Reston and blankets; avoidance of constricting wraps, straps, or tape; knee flexion; avoidance of

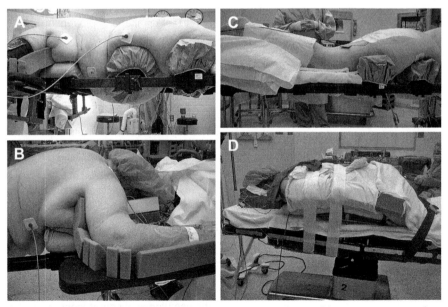

Fig. 1. Proper prone positioning of the obese patient on a spinal Jackson table. Supports are at the nipple line, anterior superior iliac spine, and proximal thigh with the panniculus and Foley catheter hanging freely (*A*). The head is in neutral position and the arms and axillae are well padded (*B*). The lower extremities are padded with Reston and the knees are flexed 20 to 30 degrees with pillows (*C*). Prone positioning for posterior subaxial spine instrumentation (*D*). (Original photographs, written permission obtained.)

shoulder hyperabduction or extension while making sure that the axillae are free; avoidance of excessive elbow flexion that stretches the ulnar nerve; and maintenance of normal cervical position. Vaidya and colleagues[10] retrospectively reviewed 63 patients with a BMI greater than 30 kg/m^2 undergoing lumbar spinal fusion. Clinical outcomes were similar to nonobese patients, but the investigators noted that blood loss, operative time, and the overall number of postoperative complications (44%) were all higher in obese patients.

Adequate exposure is more difficult in obese patients. Availability of special equipment should be ensured before starting the procedure. Extra assistants are invaluable for retraction and handling of instruments. Deep self-retaining retractors include modified cerebellars, Scoville retractors, TrimLine, and Koros retractor systems. Deep surgical fields mandate headlamps, loop or microscope magnification, and extended instruments such as long forceps and protected bovie tip extenders (**Fig. 2**).

Instrumentation and Fusion

Although it may seem intuitive that obese patients require more rigid stabilization and fusion, this remains hypothetical. Panjabi and White[28] and Panjabi and colleagues[29] discussed the effects of obesity on the spine, noting that the center of gravity shifts anteriorly. This creates a longer ventral lever arm that places more stress on the posterior tension band. Increased body weight also creates greater axial loading. Because of these factors, the surgeon should consider creating the strongest posterior construct feasible using larger pedicle screws (the pedicle may be measured on a preoperative CT scan) extending into the anterior vertebral body, increased cranial

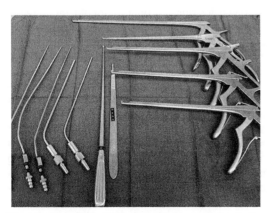

Fig. 2. Extended instrumentation useful during surgery on obese patients at all spinal levels.

and caudal extension of the construct, and meticulous fusion. Obesity has never been shown to be an independent risk factor for nonunion or pseudarthrosis after spinal fusion. Autogenous bone graft is still considered the gold standard for fusion, commonly harvested from the iliac crest (ICBG). However, complications from ICBG harvest, usually pain or dysesthesias at the harvest site, are common and well documented.[30–33] Westrich and colleagues[34] found obesity and smoking to be independent risk factors for both major and minor complications after ICBG harvest. Soft tissue complications can be minimized with careful soft tissue handling, meticulous layered closure, and drains in dead spaces to minimize hematomas. Sengupta and colleagues[35] retrospectively compared outcomes in 76 patients using local bone versus ICBG for lumbar fusion. The investigators noted decreased blood loss and length of hospital stay as well as similar fusion rates with 1-level fusion in the local bone group. However, radiographic fusion was significantly lower in multiple-level fusions in the local bone group presumably because of inadequate volume of graft. As an alternative to graft harvest, many products are available to augment posterior fusion. These bone grafting options should be reviewed by the treating surgeon with cost/benefit in mind. Bone morphogenetic protein has shown promise augmenting posterolateral fusion.[36–38] RhBMP-2 has been approved by the US Food and Drug Administration (FDA) for anterior lumbar fusion and has been studied through FDA-approved investigational device exemption (IDE) trials for posterolateral lumbar fusion. However, most cases represent off-label use based on the surgeon's individual experience and judgment.[39–42]

Postoperative Concerns

Obesity is a known risk factor for postoperative wound infection. Wimmer and colleagues[43] retrospectively reviewed 850 spinal surgeries to determine risk factors for infection. Diabetes, corticosteroid use, smoking, previous surgery, prolonged operative time, excessive blood loss, longer preoperative hospital stay, and obesity were independent risk factors. The investigators suggested that antibiotic prophylaxis be used in all posterior surgeries with consideration of extended prophylaxis if any of the these risk factors were present. There was also a lack of evidence supporting use of prophylactic antibiotics in anterior cervical surgery. Olsen and colleagues[44] performed a retrospective case-control study comparing 41 infected postoperative patients with 178 matched uninfected patients. Postoperative incontinence, posterior approach, surgery for tumor resection, and morbid obesity were independent risk factors predictive of infection following spinal surgery. Fecal incontinence increased infection risk 8-fold. Occlusive dressings and leak-proof diapers or rectal tubes are suggested. Obesity caused a fivefold increase in infections for those patients with a BMI greater than 35 kg/m^2. Increasing the dose of antibiotics (eg, 2 g of cephazolin rather than 1 g) given the poor distribution in adipose tissue as well as aggressive blood sugar control is recommended.

Spinal infections that develop in obese patients are also more difficult to treat. Only the most benign-appearing superficial infections should be treated with antibiotics and local wound care. Anything deeper or more clinically aggressive should undergo operative debridement, irrigation, and removal of loose materials such as sutures and bone graft fragments. The surgeon should obtain multiple sets of intraoperative cultures, preferably after discontinuation of antibiotics. Well-fixed hardware can remain in place except for deep aggressive infections that have proved resistant to debridement and antibiotic therapy.[45]

Minimally Invasive Surgery

When rigid fusion is necessary to ensure stability of an unstable spine, conventional open techniques should be used as outlined earlier. However, some minimally invasive techniques in lumbar spine surgery in obese patients have been shown to be safe and effective.[46,47] Early reports on minimally invasive posterior thoracolumbar instrumentation have also been promising,[48] but this type of instrumentation has not been specifically evaluated in obese patients (**Fig. 3**). This approach provides added internal

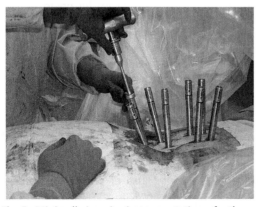

Fig. 3. Minimally invasive instrumentation of a thoracolumbar burst fracture with fluoroscopic guidance.

stabilization to a patient who may not tolerate bracing and avoids the associated morbidity of an open approach. Newer minimally invasive techniques, such as transforaminal lumbar interbody fusion and extreme lateral interbody fusion, are being increasingly used in obese patients with promising results.[46,49] Although these techniques may prove useful in treating the long-term degenerative sequelae of spinal trauma, they currently do not play a role in treating acute spinal injuries.

Wound Management

Ideal wound closure eliminates all potential dead space and creates a tight multilayered closure. Deep subfascial muscle should be loosely approximated with absorbable sutures to close dead space but not strangulate muscle leading to necrosis. Closely spaced interrupted sutures are used to close the fascial layer with care taken to close the ends of the wound. This usually necessitates an assistant to retract in the corners. Superficial Camper's fascia should next be approximated where it can be isolated. Subcutaneous sutures approximate the most superficial fat and tissue; staples or sutures are used to close the skin. The authors base drain use on the amount of anticipated draining, particularly on how much gross bleeding there was during surgery. Given the increased dead space, drains are used more frequently in the obese patient.

Postoperative Management

Medical comorbidities often necessitate postoperative admission to the ICU. This should be discussed on a case-by-case basis with the attending anesthesiologist and medical staff. Unless compelling reasons for extended prophylaxis are present (eg, open fractures, associated infections), antibiotics at increased doses should be given for only 24 hours. Upright radiographs should be obtained as a baseline to follow for progressive deformity. Prolonged immobilization increases the risks, among others, of deep vein thrombosis, respiratory complications, skin breakdown, and general deconditioning. Patients should be fitted for an orthosis, if body habitus allows, as soon as tolerated followed by aggressive mobilization and therapy. Consultation with social workers or case managers should be made early to facilitate transfer to a skilled nursing facility or an inpatient rehabilitation center. Ironically, obese patients are often medically malnourished and benefit from nutritional consultation. Despite postoperative functional improvement, lumbar spinal surgery for degenerative disease has not been shown to independently incur weight loss.[10,50]

Spinal Cord Injury Patients

With appropriate medical care and self-motivation, patients with permanent neurologic deficits from spinal cord injury can expect to live an average of 40 years after their injury.[51,52] Sixty percent of patients with spinal cord injury (SCI) are overweight or obese. The medical comorbidities associated with obesity still remain and likely become more difficult to manage. A thorough review of obesity management in patients with SCI was performed by Rajan and colleagues and published in the *Journal of Spinal Cord Medicine* in 2008.[53] The investigators stress that given the prevalence of obesity in individuals with SCI, there is an urgent need to develop practical guidelines and measures to monitor obesity in the clinical setting. They suggest that weight loss programs for individuals with SCI be designed to take into consideration the barriers to dietary and physical activity unique to this population. A potential solution in patients with such limitations may be bariatric surgery. In 2006, Alaedeen and Jasper[54] reported the first case of a successful Roux-en-Y gastric bypass in a morbidly obese paraplegic patient. Successful bariatric surgery could improve medical conditions and patient self-esteem and lessen the burden of skin care and hygiene, transfers, and transportation.

SUMMARY

Obesity is a major health epidemic. According to the available literature, obese patients involved in blunt trauma seem to incur similar spinal injuries with similar frequencies as nonobese patients. Evaluating the obese patient for spinal injury requires a thorough clinical radiographic assessment along with a high level of suspicion. Spinal injuries should be classified and treated as in nonobese patients with consideration for patient compliance and tolerance given their body habitus. Surgical intervention, particularly in the morbidly obese, may require special equipment and techniques.

Minimally invasive techniques are gaining popularity and have been useful in our experience. Thorough preoperative planning is paramount to make sure that all necessary equipment is available. Perioperative complications may be higher in obese patients, particularly infection and nerve palsies. Postoperative management should focus on close medical management, early mobilization, and weight loss strategies.

REFERENCES

1. Hedley AA, Ogden CL, Johnson CL, et al. Prevalence of overweight and obesity among US children, adolescents, and adults, 1999–2002. JAMA 2004; 291(23):2847–50.
2. Yadla S, Malone J, Campbell PG, et al. Obesity and spine surgery: reassessment based on a prospective evaluation of perioperative complications in elective degenerative thoracolumbar procedures. Spine J 2010;10(7):581–7.
3. Mangwani J, Giles C, Mullins M, et al. Obesity and recovery from low back pain: a prospective study to investigate the effect of body mass index on recovery from low back pain. Ann R Coll Surg Engl 2010;92(1):23–6.
4. Shiri R, Karppinen J, Leino-Arjas P, et al. The association between obesity and low back pain: a meta-analysis. Am J Epidemiol 2010;171(2):135–54.
5. Fanuele JC, Abdu WA, Hanscom B, et al. Association between obesity and functional status in patients with spine disease. Spine (Phila Pa 1976) 2002;27(3):306–12.
6. Telfeian AE, Reiter GT, Durham SR, et al. Spine surgery in morbidly obese patients. J Neurosurg 2002;97(Suppl 1):20–4.
7. Peltonen M, Lindroos AK, Torgerson JS. Musculoskeletal pain in the obese: a comparison with a general population and long-term changes after conventional and surgical obesity treatment. Pain 2003;104(3):549–57.
8. Mayer T, Aceska A, Gatchel RJ. Is obesity overrated as a "risk factor" for poor outcomes in chronic occupational spinal disorders? Spine (Phila Pa 1976) 2006;31(25):2967–72.
9. Patel N, Bagan B, Vadera S, et al. Obesity and spine surgery: relation to perioperative complications. J Neurosurg Spine 2007;6(4):291–7.
10. Vaidya R, Carp J, Bartol S, et al. Lumbar spine fusion in obese and morbidly obese patients. Spine (Phila Pa 1976) 2009;34(5):495–500.
11. Peng CW, Bendo JA, Goldstein JA, et al. Perioperative outcomes of anterior lumbar surgery in obese versus non-obese patients. Spine J 2009;9(9):715–20.
12. Young T, Peppard PE, Taheri S. Excess weight and sleep-disordered breathing. J Appl Physiol 2005; 99(4):1592–9.
13. Eckert DJ, Malhotra A. Pathophysiology of adult obstructive sleep apnea. Proc Am Thorac Soc 2008;5(2):144–53.
14. Teran-Santos J, Jimenez-Gomez A, Cordero-Guevara J. The association between sleep apnea and the risk of traffic accidents. Cooperative Group Burgos-Santander. N Engl J Med 1999;340(11):847–51.
15. Findley LJ, Unverzagt ME, Suratt PM. Automobile accidents involving patients with obstructive sleep apnea. Am Rev Respir Dis 1988;138(2):337–40.

16. Brown CV, Neville AL, Rhee P, et al. The impact of obesity on the outcomes of 1,153 critically injured blunt trauma patients. J Trauma 2005;59(5): 1048–51 [discussion: 1051].

17. Boulanger BR, Milzman D, Mitchell K, et al. Body habitus as a predictor of injury pattern after blunt trauma. J Trauma 1992;33(2):228–32.

18. Ravi B, Rampersaud R. Clinical magnification error in lateral spinal digital radiographs. Spine (Phila Pa 1976) 2008;33(10):E311–6.

19. Como JJ, Diaz JJ, Dunham CM, et al. Practice management guidelines for identification of cervical spine injuries following trauma: update from the Eastern Association for the Surgery of Trauma Practice Management Guidelines Committee. J Trauma 2009;67(3):651–9.

20. Ginde AA, Foianini A, Renner DM, et al. The challenge of CT and MRI imaging of obese individuals who present to the emergency department: a national survey. Obesity (Silver Spring) 2008; 16(11):2549–51.

21. Vaccaro AR, et al. A new classification of thoracolumbar injuries: the importance of injury morphology, the integrity of the posterior ligamentous complex, and neurologic status. Spine (Phila Pa 1976) 2005; 30(20):2325–33.

22. Vaccaro AR, et al. The subaxial cervical spine injury classification system: a novel approach to recognize the importance of morphology, neurology, and integrity of the disco-ligamentous complex. Spine (Phila Pa 1976) 2007;32(21):2365–74.

23. Kroonen LT, Herman M, Pizzutillo PD, et al. Prader-Willi syndrome: clinical concerns for the orthopaedic surgeon. J Pediatr Orthop 2006;26(5):673–9.

24. O'Neill PJ, Karol LA, Shindle MK, et al. Decreased orthotic effectiveness in overweight patients with adolescent idiopathic scoliosis. J Bone Joint Surg Am 2005;87(5):1069–74.

25. Goodkin R, Laska LL. Wrong disc space level surgery: medicolegal implications. Surg Neurol 2004;61(4):323–41 [discussion: 341–2].

26. Roh MS, Wilson-Holden TJ, Padberg AM, et al. The utility of somatosensory evoked potential monitoring during cervical spine surgery: how often does it prompt intervention and affect outcome? Asian Spine J 2007;1(1):43–7.

27. Brodsky JB, Oldroyd M, Winfield HN, et al. Morbid obesity and the prone position: a case report. J Clin Anesth 2001;13(2):138–40.

28. Panjabi MM, White AA 3rd. Basic biomechanics of the spine. Neurosurgery 1980;7(1):76–93.

29. Panjabi MM, Thibodeau LL, Crisco JJ 3rd, et al. What constitutes spinal instability? Clin Neurosurg 1988;34:313–39.

30. Banwart JC, Asher MA, Hassanein RS. Iliac crest bone graft harvest donor site morbidity. A statistical evaluation. Spine (Phila Pa 1976) 1995;20(9): 1055–60.

31. Younger EM, Chapman MW. Morbidity at bone graft donor sites. J Orthop Trauma 1989;3(3):192–5.

32. Arrington ED, Smith WJ, Chambers HG, et al. Complications of iliac crest bone graft harvesting. Clin Orthop Relat Res 1996;329:300–9.

33. Fernyhough JC, Schimandle JJ, Weigel MC, et al. Chronic donor site pain complicating bone graft harvesting from the posterior iliac crest for spinal fusion. Spine (Phila Pa 1976) 1992;17(12):1474–80.

34. Westrich GH, Geller DS, O'Malley MJ, et al. Anterior iliac crest bone graft harvesting using the cortico-cancellous reamer system. J Orthop Trauma 2001; 15(7):500–6.

35. Sengupta DK, Truumees E, Patel CK, et al. Outcome of local bone versus autogenous iliac crest bone graft in the instrumented posterolateral fusion of the lumbar spine. Spine (Phila Pa 1976) 2006; 31(9):985–91.

36. Mulconrey DS, Bridwell KH, Flynn J, et al. Bone morphogenetic protein (RhBMP-2) as a substitute for iliac crest bone graft in multilevel adult spinal deformity surgery: minimum two-year evaluation of fusion. Spine (Phila Pa 1976) 2008;33(20):2153–9.

37. Luhmann SJ, Bridwell KH, Cheng I, et al. Use of bone morphogenetic protein-2 for adult spinal deformity. Spine (Phila Pa 1976) 2005;30(17 Suppl): S110–7.

38. Kraiwattanapong C, Boden SD, Louis-Ugbo J, et al. Comparison of Healos/bone marrow to INFUSE (rhBMP-2/ACS) with a collagen-ceramic sponge bulking agent as graft substitutes for lumbar spine fusion. Spine (Phila Pa 1976) 2005;30(9):1001–7 [discussion: 1007].

39. Carreon LY, Glassman SD, Djurasovic M, et al. RhBMP-2 versus iliac crest bone graft for lumbar spine fusion in patients over 60 years of age: a cost-utility study. Spine (Phila Pa 1976) 2009; 34(3):238–43.

40. Glassman SD, Dimar JR 3rd, Burkus K, et al. The efficacy of rhBMP-2 for posterolateral lumbar fusion in smokers. Spine (Phila Pa 1976) 2007;32(15): 1693–8.

41. Glassman SD, Carreon LY, Djurasovic M, et al. RhBMP-2 versus iliac crest bone graft for lumbar spine fusion: a randomized, controlled trial in patients over sixty years of age. Spine (Phila Pa 1976) 2008;33(26):2843–9.

42. Dimar JR 2nd, Glassman SD, Burkus JK, et al. Clinical and radiographic analysis of an optimized rhBMP-2 formulation as an autograft replacement in posterolateral lumbar spine arthrodesis. J Bone Joint Surg Am 2009;91(6):1377–86.

43. Wimmer C, Gluch H, Franzreb M, et al. Predisposing factors for infection in spine surgery: a survey of 850

spinal procedures. J Spinal Disord 1998;11(2): 124–8.

44. Olsen MA, Nepple JJ, Riew KD, et al. Risk factors for surgical site infection following orthopaedic spinal operations. J Bone Joint Surg Am 2008;90(1):62–9.

45. Beiner JM, Grauer J, Kwon BK, et al. Postoperative wound infections of the spine. Neurosurg Focus 2003;15(3):E14.

46. Park P, Upadhyaya C, Garton HJ, et al. The impact of minimally invasive spine surgery on perioperative complications in overweight or obese patients. Neurosurgery 2008;62(3):693–9 [discussion: 693–9].

47. Tomasino A, Parikh K, Steinberger J, et al. Tubular microsurgery for lumbar discectomies and laminectomies in obese patients: operative results and outcome. Spine (Phila Pa 1976) 2009;34(18): E664–72.

48. Wild MH, Glees M, Plieschnegger C, et al. Five-year follow-up examination after purely minimally invasive posterior stabilization of thoracolumbar fractures: a comparison of minimally invasive percutaneously and conventionally open treated patients. Arch Orthop Trauma Surg 2007;127(5): 335–43.

49. Rodgers WB, et al. Early complications of extreme lateral interbody fusion in the obese. J Spinal Disord 2010;23(6):393–7.

50. Garcia RM, Messerschmitt PJ, Furey CG, et al. Weight loss in overweight and obese patients following successful lumbar decompression. J Bone Joint Surg Am 2008;90(4):742–7.

51. DeVivo MJ, Go BK, Jackson AB. Overview of the national spinal cord injury statistical center database. J Spinal Cord Med 2002;25(4):335–8.

52. DeVivo M, Biering-Sorensen F, Charlifue S, et al. International spinal cord injury core data set. Spinal Cord 2006;44(9):535–40.

53. Rajan S, McNeely MJ, Warms C, et al. Clinical assessment and management of obesity in individuals with spinal cord injury: a review. J Spinal Cord Med 2008;31(4):361–72.

54. Alaedeen DI, Jasper J. Gastric bypass surgery in a paraplegic morbidly obese patient. Obes Surg 2006;16(8):1107–8.

Obesity in Pediatric Orthopaedics

F. Keith Gettys, MD, J. Benjamin Jackson, MD,
Steven L. Frick, MD*

KEYWORDS

- Obesity • Pediatric • Tibia vara
- Slipped capital femoral epiphysis

Obesity is a rapidly expanding health problem in children and adolescents, and is the most prevalent nutritional problem for children in the United States. In addition to poor nutrition, sedentary activity is a significant contributor to childhood obesity. The many reasons for lower physical activity levels in today's youth include time spent watching television or at a computer, not walking or riding to school, cutting back on school physical education programs, and increasing use of labor-saving mechanical devices. Some believe that obesity has become a major epidemic in American children, with the prevalence having more than doubled since 1980.[1–3] The combination of genetic and environmental factors contributing to increasing levels of obese children and the roles of insulin excess and leptin resistance are nicely reviewed in articles by Lustig and colleagues.[4–6] As in adults, Body Mass Index (BMI) has been used to screen for overweight and obese patients. BMI is defined as kilograms per meter squared, representing a function of body weight and height. It is adjusted for age and gender and is subdivided into BMI percentiles.[7] In children and adolescents, a BMI in the 85th to 95th percentile or a BMI of 25–30 kg/m^2 is considered overweight, whereas a child above the 95th percentile or with a BMI greater than 30 kg/m^2 is considered obese.[8,9] This epidemic has led to a near-doubling in hospitalizations with a diagnosis of obesity between 1999 and 2005 and an increase in costs from $125.9 million to 237.6 million between 2001 and 2005.[10]

Childhood obesity has a well-documented association with multiple medical comorbidities.[7,11,12] Additionally, children that are overweight are more likely to become overweight adults than their normal-weight peers.[11,13–16] Obesity in adulthood has been linked to many diseases, including cardiovascular disease, type 2 diabetes mellitus, osteoarthritis, chronic back pain, and obstructive sleep apnea.[12]

This article describes some of the orthopaedic conditions commonly encountered in overweight/obese children and adolescents, classically infantile and adolescent tibia vara and slipped capital femoral epiphysis (SCFE). Also discussed are genu valgum, which has also been associated with obesity, and other difficulties encountered in providing orthopaedic care to obese children.

MUSCULOSKELETAL TRAUMA IN OBESE PEDIATRIC PATIENTS

Pediatric patients most commonly seek orthopaedic care for musculoskeletal trauma, and most fractures in childhood are treated with closed methods. Maintaining correct alignment and positioning using splints or casts relies on the principles of 3-point contact and proper molding. The large soft-tissue envelope of obese children can make safe and secure casting difficult, potentially leading to skin complications, to loss of fracture reduction, and to a decision to treat injuries operatively rather than with casting. When surgery is planned, the greater loads across the fracture in obese patients may require more rigid fixation than is typically used in pediatric patients.

In the adult population, obesity has been found to be an independent risk factor of trauma-related morbidity, although there is a decreased risk of

The authors have nothing to disclose.
Department of Orthopaedic Surgery, Carolinas Medical Center, PO Box 32861, Charlotte, NC 28232, USA
* Corresponding author.
E-mail address: steven.frick@carolinashealthcare.org

Orthop Clin N Am 42 (2011) 95–105
doi:10.1016/j.ocl.2010.08.005

orthopedic.theclinics.com

fractures. However, a chart review and question-naire study performed by Taylor and colleagues[17] noted that overweight children had a higher incidence of fractures. They also found a higher incidence of musculoskeletal pain, specifically knee pain. Skaggs and colleagues[18] found that girls who sustained forearm fractures from a low-energy mechanism were more likely to be obese, with a radius that had a decreased cross-sectional area when compared with matched controls without forearm fractures. It was proposed that the smaller cross-sectional diameter combined with increased body mass and minor trauma created a predisposition to fracture in these patients.

Others studies have questioned the reasons for increased numbers of fractures in the obese adolescent population. Leonard and colleagues[19] and Taylor and colleagues[17] found increased bone mineral density in obese adolescents, although the relationship of bone mass to obesity is controversial and often conflicting. These findings have led some to propose that the increased risk of fracture is due to the inactivity that contributes to obesity. Inactivity may lead to decreased proprioception and poor balance, leading to an increased risk of falling.

When fractures do occur in the obese, complications are increased. Rana and colleagues[20] examined the effect of obesity on numerous outcome measures at their level 1 trauma center. They found that obese children had an increased incidence of extremity fractures, fractures necessitating operative intervention, decubitus ulcers, and deep venous thrombosis (DVT). The findings of increased DVT were confirmed in a study by Vu and colleagues[21] examining the risk factors of DVT in hospitalized children, which found that obesity was a risk factor with a prevalence ratio of 2.1. Literature on adults suggests that obesity may be a risk factor of venous thromboembolic disease (VTED). VTED is fortunately rare in children who do not have coagulopathies, and this rarity leads to controversy about the appropriateness of chemoprophylaxis in pediatric patients, especially in adolescents approaching skeletal maturity/adulthood. Not enough data is available to make recommendations about the value or efficacy of VTED prophylaxis in obese adolescents.

Leet and colleagues[22] found that obese children (BMI >95th percentile) and *extremely heavy* children (BMI between the 90th and 94th percentile) with operatively treated femur fractures had a significantly increased incidence of complications. The complications included: refracture, pin-site infection requiring debridement, loss of alignment in frame, wound infection, malunion,

osteomyelitis, wound dehiscence, compartment syndrome, broken rod, and broken pin. Fracture stabilization must be augmented in the obese patient, because of the known limitations and increased incidence of implant failure. Recent studies of titanium elastic nails used for pediatric femur fractures has found an increased incidence of malunion in children weighing more than 45 kg. Several studies have found that weight was an independent risk factor of malunion.[23–25] Some have suggested that patients weighing more than 45.36 kg should undergo intramedullary nail fixation using small diameter nails with interlocking screws. The key with any of these devices is to enter the femur though the trochanter, not the piriformis fossa, and not to cross the distal femoral epiphysis with the implant. Another fixation option that is more rigid than elastic nailing is plate fixation, with open or submuscular approaches.[26]

If operative treatment is chosen, obesity can alter physiologic responses to surgical procedures. Studies indicate that obese adults undergoing surgical procedures have an increased risk of complications, and the actual procedures are technically more challenging because of their body mass.[27] The senior author's experience is that musculoskeletal procedures to stabilize fractures or perform osteotomies in obese pediatric patients are technically more difficult, involving positioning challenges, difficulties obtaining adequate intraoperative imaging, larger incisions, longer operative times, and more complications.

Few studies are available to evaluate the impact of childhood obesity on surgical procedures. A retrospective review of pediatric surgical patients over a 4-year period found increased preoperative diagnoses of medical comorbidities and prolonged recovery room stays in obese children compared with normal-weight children.[27] Davies and Yanchar[28] found that obese children undergoing appendectomies had problems before, during, and after surgery that were similar to those experienced by obese adults. An increased use of sophisticated scanning suggested that appendicitis is difficult to diagnose in obese children. Additionally, they found that childhood obesity led to increased surgical times, increased risk of wound infections, and increased time to ambulation.

The difficulties noted earlier also translate to orthopaedic practice. Obese children presenting for orthopaedic evaluation may prove more difficult to manage, because physical examinations to identify joint effusions, joint laxity, and soft tissue masses are more difficult when the extremities have a thick layer of subcutaneous fat. Operative procedures on the lower extremities in obese children can substantially impair mobility, because the children often do not have sufficient upper extremity strength to ambulate safely with crutches or a walker. Postoperative respiratory difficulties may be exacerbated by poor mobilization.

Similar to adults, obstructive sleep apnea (OSA) is a comorbidity that warrants consideration in children, because it can increase the risks of anesthesia during a surgical procedure. OSA can lead to nocturnal snoring, hypoxia, and hypercarbia and has a prevalence of 2% in children. [29] OSA has been associated with increased perioperative anesthetic complications, including difficulty with intubation and acute respiratory failure during the induction of anesthesia. Additionally, postoperative complications have been reported, including hypoxia, airway edema, obstruction of the upper airway, pulmonary edema, and respiratory failure. Gordon and colleagues[29] reported that 11 of 18 patients with Blount disease who were older than 9 years had been diagnosed with sleep apnea and required noninvasive positive-pressure ventilation. The orthopaedic surgeon should ask obese adolescents about snoring as a risk factor of OSA and take appropriate supportive measures before, during, and after surgery.

EFFECTS OF OBESITY ON THE GROWING SKELETON

Several common orthopaedic clinical situations in overweight children are created by increased mechanical load on growing bones. Bone is a dynamic tissue that responds to the mechanical stresses and loads placed on it. The differentiating factor in pediatric orthopaedics is that the bones are growing, and the growth plate is a specialized organ that is also sensitive to the surrounding mechanical environment. Two laws or principles have long been offered to explain the effects of mechanical loading on the longitudinal growth of bone.[30] The Hueter-Volkmann law states that bone growth is suppressed by an additional compressive loading through the immature growth plate, and growth is accelerated by reduced loading.[30,31] Similarly, the Delpech law states that increasing tension across the growth plate leads to increased growth. [30,31] These laws describe complex physiologic relationships, the mechanisms of which have been studied but are not completely understood.[32]

The Hueter-Volkmann and Delpech laws can explain some of the pathologic conditions related to the increased loading of growth plates in the overweight child. Several basic science experiments have found that static, sustained loads affect growth plates in different animals, with increased compression leading to reduced longitudinal growth.[32–35] Similarly, although not as well defined, when tension was applied across the growth plate in lambs, they experienced an increase in growth.[33] Applying the Hueter-Volkmann theory to overweight children, the additional weight on their growth plates could lead to an increased load or compression, creating a decrease in growth, especially on the concavity of a malaligned joint (example medial knee joint in genu varum). Conversely, if there is malalignment of a load-bearing joint leading to tensile forces across the convexity of the joint (eg,the lateral knee joint in genu varum), those distraction forces may lead to less pressure across the physis and accelerated growth (Delpech law). Thus a vicious cycle is established, in which malalignment leads to abnormal mechanical forces creating abnormal physeal growth, causing worsening malalignment. Biopsy studies of the 3 pediatric orthopaedic conditions (infantile tibia vara, adolescent tibia vara, and SCFE), commonly believed to be related to obesity and resultant mechanical overload of the physis, have demonstrated histopathology findings supportive of this hypothesis.[36–38] Abnormal forces are thought to disrupt physeal growth and suppress endochondral ossification, leading to deformities. Others have noted that similar pathophysiology may be involved in genu valgum and scoliosis deformities.

The Knee

The knee is the most common site of musculoskeletal pain in overweight children.[17] The knee's position and overall alignment are critical when assessing the effects of increased weight on an overweight child. Two conditions, genu varum and genu valgum, involving the knee joint in children have been linked to obesity, with higher overall incidences in the overweight population.

Blount Disease or Tibia Vara

Blount disease is a developmental disorder involving abnormal growth from the medial part of the proximal tibial physis. It was first described by Blount[39] in 1937 as only a frontal plane deformity(tibia vara), but subsequently, other authors have noted that multiplanar deformities are commonly seen.[40,41] Abnormal, asymmetric growth results in a 3-dimensional deformity of the tibia with primarily varus, procurvatum, and internal rotation (**Fig. 1**).[42]

These deformities have been shown to lead to progressive deformity, with gait deviations, limb-length discrepancy, and premature arthritis of the knee.[42–45] There are 2 clinically distinct forms of Blount disease, infantile and adolescent, which

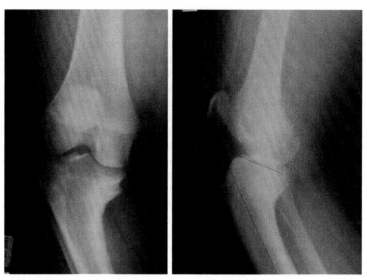

Fig. 1. Radiographs of a patient with Blount disease. One can see 3 characteristic deformities: tibia vara, internal tibial rotation, and procurvatum. (*Courtesy of* George V. Russell, MD, University of Mississippi Medical Center, MS, USA.)

are based on whether the limb deformity develops before or after age 4 years.[46] The exact cause of both forms of Blount disease has yet to be fully determined. Many have suggested a mechanical basis for the disease, based on the observations that the disease occurs more frequently in children who start walking at an early age and those who are overweight.[46–50] Blount disease has long been associated with increased weight and obesity.[42,51,52]

The deformity to the proximal tibia is thought to be due to excessive medial compressive forces causing growth inhibition (Heuter-Volkman law).[42] In a child with genu varum, obesity has been shown to substantially increase the compressive forces created on the medial compartment of the knee.[47,49,50] Cook and colleagues[47] assessed the load distribution in the proximal tibia as a function of varus or valgus alignment, and they estimated physeal growth inhibition by applied compression forces. They determined that 20° of varus deformity in an obese 2-year-old and 10° of varus deformity in an obese 5-year-old could generate enough compressive force to retard growth of the medial tibial physis. In another study, Dietz and colleagues[49] looked at the relationship between the percentage of ideal body weight and the tibiofemoral shaft angles. They found a significant correlation ($r = 0.75$) with a mixture of obese and nonobese patients; however, they found a stronger correlation ($r = 0.90$) among the obese only. The effect of childhood obesity on 3-dimensional knee biomechanics was studied by Gushue and colleagues[50] using gait analysis. Overweight children showed substantially higher

peak internal knee abduction moments during early stance with increased loading of the medial compartment of the knee joint compared with children of normal weight, potentially contributing to development of varus alignment.

Infantile Blount disease affects children before age 4 years. Bilateral involvement is common and more likely to occur in the infantile form.[46] The infantile form affects girls and boys equally; however, African American children are affected more commonly than other children.[53] Infantile Blount disease develops between the ages of 2 and 4 years, when normal physiologic varus seen in infants progresses to physiologic valgus, and it must be distinguished from physiologic bowing.[54] Scott and colleagues[52] compared children with physiologic bowing and those diagnosed with infantile Blount disease and found a significantly increased BMI in those with infantile Blount disease. Sabharwal and colleagues[42] found that the infantile form had more severe varus and procurvatum deformities of the proximal tibia than did those with the adolescent form. They also found that the magnitude of deformity strongly correlated with increased weight in those with the early form of the disease and that the correlation with deformity was stronger in extremely obese individuals (BMI >40) (**Fig. 2**). The authors of one paper thought that the greater deformity in the younger patients was due to the differences in the epiphyses due to aging.[38] They proposed that there was increased pliability in the unossified epiphyses of younger patients, leading to more growth inhibition than in adolescents. These findings support the development of the deformity being

A B

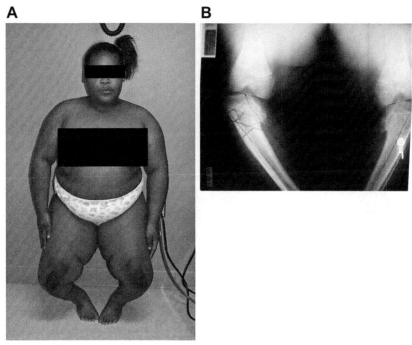

Fig. 2. (*A*) Clinical image of a morbidly obese young girl with severe Blount disease. The child's deformity was so severe that she was unable to walk any considerable distance. Close inspection shows skin thickening over her patellae secondary to her need to crawl for short-range ambulation, otherwise she required a wheelchair (*Courtesy of* George V. Russell, MD, University of Mississippi Medical Center, MS, USA.) (*B*) Radiographs of patient shown in **Fig. 2**A. Note the marked tibia vara and the associated articular malformation of the proximal tibia, particularly the medial aspect.

attributed to abnormal loading of the proximal tibial physis.

Adolescent Blount disease is less common than the infantile form, and the incidence is higher in the male sex; yet, African Americans who are morbidly obese comprise more than 90% of the reported cases.[48] One study found the prevalence of adolescent Blount disease to be 2.5% in obese male adolescents.[55] There were theories that the adolescent form was due to massive weight gain during adolescence in individuals with underlying varus alignment that could lead to excessive medial compartment loading and altered physeal growth (**Fig. 3**A).[48] However, one observational study found no correlation between varus static alignment and development of the adolescent form.[56] Along these lines, Davids and colleagues[48] examined the gait deviations related to the increased thigh girth associated with adolescent obesity. Their hypothesis was that obese children with larger thighs would have difficulty adequately adducting their hips and this could result in "fat-thigh" gait. They concluded that a fat-thigh gait could produce a varus moment at the knee, leading to increased compressive forces at the medial part of the proximal tibial physis sufficient to retard physeal

growth (**Fig. 4**). Although data suggest that obesity may lead to excessive loading of the proximal medial tibial physis, it is unlikely that this is the sole cause of the deformity.

For both forms of Blount disease, the treatment is customized based on the child's age, the magnitude of the deformity, the limb-length discrepancy, the psychosocial factors, and the surgeon's experience.[46] Nonoperative modalities for infantile Blount disease include orthoses or surgical management. Once Blount disease is diagnosed, progressive deformity is expected and observation is not recommended. The natural history of significant varus malalignment of the knee is early medial compartment osteoarthrosis, leading pediatric orthopaedic surgeons to attempt to normalize coronal plane alignment with orthotic or surgical treatment. The guiding treatment principle is to decrease the compressive forces acting on the medial physeal region, to allow the reversal of pathologic processes and restore normal growth.[57] Surgical treatment options include various types of realignment osteotomies, guided growth, gradual asymmetrical physeal distraction, resection of a physeal bar, and elevation of the medial tibial plateau. The indications and descriptions of these techniques

A   **B**

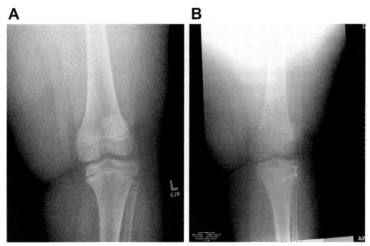

Fig. 3. (*A*) An obese 12-year-old boy with unilateral tibia vara and characteristic physeal abnormalities. (*B*) Growth modulation with lateral tension band plates can often correct the mechanical axis deviation if the patient has enough growth remaining. In patients with very fat thighs, as seen here, some residual varus alignment may be desired to prevent the thighs from rubbing together during gait and to keep them from pushing the knees and feet too far laterally.

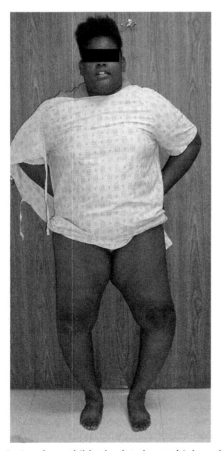

Fig. 4. An obese child who has large thighs, which may have contributed to a "fat-thigh" gait and subsequent tibia vara. (*Courtesy of* George V. Russell, MD, University of Mississippi Medical Center, MS, USA.)

are beyond the scope of this article; however, the specific literature related to surgery and overweight patients is reviewed.

Pirpiris and colleagues[51] observed children requiring surgery for the treatment of infantile and late-onset Blount disease and found a clear relationship of increased surgery with increased BMI. For the adolescent form of Blount disease, there are no effective nonoperative treatments for substantial degrees of adolescent tibia vara. If the patient has substantial growth remaining, a guided growth strategy can be effective and can avoid the potential morbidity of osteotomies. McIntosh and colleagues[58] found that BMI of more than 45 kg/m^2 was a risk factor of failure of lateral hemiepiphysiodesis in the treatment of adolescent tibia vara. One of the guided growth techniques uses a tension band plate on the convex side of the growth plate (see **Fig. 3**B). The implant chosen for this method of correction might require consideration of the patient's weight and body habitus. Schroerlucke and colleagues[59] reported 8 failures out of 31 patients with their use of 8-plate tension band device treatment of angular deformities. All 8 failures were in patients with Blount disease, with an unacceptable failure rate of 44%. They concluded that stronger plates need to be used in Blount disease. Some have recommended 2 adjacent plates in the heavier adolescents to decrease implant failure.[46] Stanitski and colleagues[60] reported on the use of the Ilizarov circular external fixator, with gradual correction of 17 obese patients with adolescent tibia vara. The only complications were one delayed union and one premature consolidation; however, all achieved alignment within 5° of normal. They concluded that in this high risk surgical patient population, circular external fixation was an excellent treatment method. Others have noted substantial difficulty in achieving surgical alignment goals using unilateral external fixation, with frequent complications.[61] Complications including wound healing problems, infections, pin tract sepsis, nerve palsies, and compartment syndrome have been reported.

Genu Valgum

Obesity may also predispose the knee to the development of a valgus deformity. Genu valgum is most commonly physiologic and requires no surgical intervention.[62,63] Pathologic causes of genu valgum have been described after fractures with certain hereditary disorders and associated with infectious and metabolic disorders.[63] Although limited data link obesity to genu valgum, the theory is that in children and adolescents who have valgus alignment at the knee, increased weight leads to greater compression on the lateral distal femoral physis (Hueter-Volkmann law), leading to diminished lateral growth and progressive valgus deformity (**Fig. 5**). Zhang and colleagues[64] described 2 cases of overweight girls without a history of prior injury or medical

condition who developed progressive genu valgum. They proposed that obesity led to repetitive microtrauma at the distal femoral physis, contributing to the deformity. Stevens and colleagues[62] also found a correlation of obesity and valgus deformity of the knee in a gait analysis study. Of the 16 patients studied, six (37.5%) were obese, showing a correlation of increased weight or BMI to genu valgum. Their study showed that genu valgum could predispose to abnormal knee joint kinetics, including increased knee valgus, increased hip abduction, and frontal plane knee moments. Finally, they suggested that early recognition of potentially progressive valgus deformity of the knee may allow for earlier correction and restoration of lower extremity biomechanics.

SCFE

SCFE is a condition in which the proximal femoral metaphysis separates from the epiphysis of the femoral head. This condition usually occurs during the most rapid growth phase of adolescence, typically between age 11 and 15 years. The exact cause of the disease is unknown, but numerous studies have identified risk factors including obesity, increased femoral retroversion, pituitary axis disorders, and endocrinopathies. SCFE is usually diagnosed in ambulatory patients when radiographs are ordered for long-standing knee,

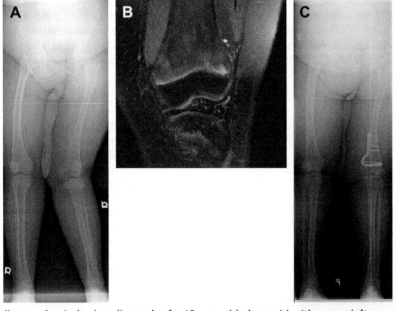

Fig. 5. (*A*) Standing mechanical axis radiograph of a 12-year-old obese girl with severe left genu valgum associated with irregular physes as described by Zhang. (*B*) Magnetic resonance imaging demonstrates abnormal cartilage protrusions into the metaphysis in areas of physeal widening. Zhang proposed that these changes were the result of abnormal loading of the physis. (*C*) Corrective distal femoral osteotomy with blade plate fixation was used to restore more normal limb alignment.

hip, or thigh pain, or to evaluate a limp. There is usually no specific history of trauma, although occasionally, patients present with inability to bear weight after an acute event. These cases often have a history of antecedent groin, hip, or knee pain, because SCFE is believed to develop slowly and not purely as the result of an acute traumatic episode (**Fig. 6**).

Manoff[65] found that 81% of patients diagnosed with an SCFE had a BMI greater than or equal to the 95th percentile. Bhatia and colleagues[66] examined the risk factors of bilateral disease or progression to bilateral disease. They found that children with bilateral disease on presentation had a significantly higher BMI. They also found that children who presented with unilateral disease but progressed to bilateral disease had a significantly increased BMI. In their population, every child with a BMI greater than 35 kg/m^2 eventually had bilateral disease.

Obesity in this population has been found to lead to other biomechanical risk factors of the disease. Obese adolescents have increased femoral retroversion of approximately 10° in the affected an unaffected sides. Studies have also examined obese and nonobese controls and found that obese children had increased retroversion of the femoral neck. Obese adolescents also have an increased physeal slope and a deeper acetabular socket or center-edge angle. Each of these 3findings linked to childhood obesity lead to increased stress on the femoral physis and create a favorable environment for SCFE.[67–69]

Two studies have found a correlation between increased prevalence of childhood obesity and increased incidence of SCFE. In their Scottish population, Murray and Wilson[70] found a correlation between obesity and SCFE. They found that the incidence of SCFE has risen from 3.78 per 100,000 in 1981 to 9.66 per 100,000 in 2000. They noted that during this same period, the age of presentation of SCFE had decreased in both boys and girls. They further noted that from 1981 to 2005, the number of severely obese children had quadrupled and the number of overweight children aged between 13 and 15 years had nearly tripled. Benson and colleagues[71] found a correlation between increased obesity and disease prevalence in New Mexico. They examined the incidence of the disease from 1995 to 2006. During the 1960s, the incidence of SCFE was 2.13 per 100,000 children in the state of New Mexico; however, during the study period, the incidence had risen to 5.99 per 100,000. They also noted an increase in the incidence of 2.27 cases per 100,000 from the start of the study in 1995 to 1997 to 7.38 cases per 100,000 between 2004 and 2006. Coincidentally, from 1971 to 2004, the National Health and Nutrition Examination Survey found New Mexico's rate of obesity had tripled.

As the incidence of childhood obesity is increasing, so too is the incidence of SCFE. This should increase the clinician's suspicion in the obese child with knee, thigh, or hip pain with or without antecedent trauma. The data for prophylactic pinning of the contralateral hip in very overweight or obese patients is not clear, because studies looking at the risk of a subsequent contralateral slip have not analyzed weight or BMI independently as a risk factor.[72] Bilateral disease is more prevalent in very obese patients, and perhaps that should be a consideration when deciding whether or not prophylactic pinning is indicated.[73,74]

SUMMARY

Obesity is an increasing problem for children and adolescents in much of the world, but particularly in the United States. Orthopaedic surgeons will be confronted with much in the way of musculoskeletal difficulties and pathologies related to obesity. Hopefully, new programs that address childhood nutritional and activity issues can reverse the worrying trends of increasing obesity.[9,75,76] In the mean time, orthopaedic surgeons must focus their efforts on effectively diagnosing and treating this growing segment of the population.

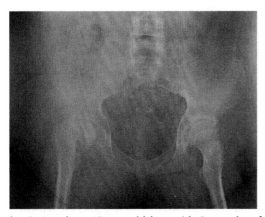

Fig. 6. An obese 13-year-old boy with 2 months of antecedent knee pain, presenting with an unstable right SCFE. Note the large abdominal soft tissue shadow on the radiograph.

REFERENCES

1. Ogden CL, Carroll MD, Curtin LR, et al. Prevalence of high body mass index in US children and adolescents, 2007–2008. JAMA 2010;303(3):242–9.

2. Ogden CL, Carroll MD, Flegal KM. High body mass index for age among US children and adolescents, 2003–2006. JAMA 2008;299(20):2401–5.

3. Ogden CL, Flegal KM, Carroll MD, et al. Prevalence and trends in overweight among US children and adolescents, 1999–2000. JAMA 2002;288(14):1728–32.

4. Jasik CB, Lustig RH. Adolescent obesity and puberty: the "perfect storm". Ann N Y Acad Sci 2008;1135:265–79.

5. Lustig RH. Which comes first? The obesity or the insulin? The behavior or the biochemistry? J Pediatr 2008;152(5):601–2.

6. Mietus-Snyder ML, Lustig RH. Childhood obesity: adrift in the "limbic triangle". Annu Rev Med 2008; 59:147–62.

7. Dietz WH. Health consequences of obesity in youth: childhood predictors of adult disease. Pediatrics 1998;101(3 Pt 2):518–25.

8. Barlow SE, Dietz WH. Obesity evaluation and treatment: expert Committee recommendations. The Maternal and child health bureau, health resources and services administration and the department of health and human services. Pediatrics 1998; 102(3):E29.

9. Krebs NF, Jacobson MS. Prevention of pediatric overweight and obesity. Pediatrics 2003;112(2): 424–30.

10. Trasande L, Liu Y, Fryer G, et al. Effects of childhood obesity on hospital care and costs, 1999–2005. Health Aff (Millwood) 2009;28(4):w751–60.

11. Guo SS, Wu W, Chumlea WC, et al. Predicting overweight and obesity in adulthood from body mass index values in childhood and adolescence. Am J Clin Nutr 2002;76(3):653–8.

12. Visscher TL, Seidell JC. The public health impact of obesity. Annu Rev Public Health 2001;22:355–75.

13. Eriksson J, Forsen T, Osmond C, et al. Obesity from cradle to grave. Int J Obes Relat Metab Disord 2003; 27(6):722–7.

14. Gunturu SD, Ten S. Complications of obesity in childhood. Pediatr Ann 2007;36(2):96–101.

15. Serdula MK, Ivery D, Coates RJ, et al. Do obese children become obese adults? A review of the literature. Prev Med 1993;22(2):167–77.

16. Whitaker RC, Wright JA, Pepe MS, et al. Predicting obesity in young adulthood from childhood and parental obesity. N Engl J Med 1997;337(13): 869–73.

17. Taylor ED, Theim KR, Mirch MC, et al. Orthopedic complications of overweight in children and adolescents. Pediatrics 2006;117(6):2167–74.

18. Skaggs DL, Loro ML, Pitukcheewanont P, et al. Increased body weight and decreased radial cross-sectional dimensions in girls with forearm fractures. J Bone Miner Res 2001;16(7):1337–42.

19. Leonard MB, Shults J, Wilson BA, et al. Obesity during childhood and adolescence augments bone mass and bone dimensions. Am J Clin Nutr 2004; 80(2):514–23.

20. Rana AR, Michalsky MP, Teich S, et al. Childhood obesity: a risk factor for injuries observed at a level-1 trauma center. J Pediatr Surg 2009;44(8): 1601–5.

21. Vu LT, Nobuhara KK, Lee H, et al. Determination of risk factors for deep venous thrombosis in hospitalized children. J Pediatr Surg 2008;43(6):1095–9.

22. Leet AI, Pichard CP, Ain MC. Surgical treatment of femoral fractures in obese children: does excessive body weight increase the rate of complications? J Bone Joint Surg Am 2005;87(12):2609–13.

23. Mehlman CT, Bishai SK. Tibial nails for femoral shaft fractures in large adolescents with open femoral physes. J Trauma 2007;63(2):424–8.

24. Moroz LA, Launay F, Kocher MS, et al. Titanium elastic nailing of fractures of the femur in children. Predictors of complications and poor outcome. J Bone Joint Surg Br 2006;88(10):1361–6.

25. Weiss JM, Choi P, Ghatan C, et al. Complications with flexible nailing of femur fractures more than double with child obesity and weight >50 kg. J Child Orthop 2009;3(1):53–8.

26. Kuremsky MA, Frick SL. Advances in the surgical management of pediatric femoral shaft fractures. Curr Opin Pediatr 2007;19(1):51–7.

27. Nafiu OO, Ndao-Brumlay KS, Bamgbade OA, et al. Prevalence of overweight and obesity in a U.S. pediatric surgical population. J Natl Med Assoc 2007; 99(1):46–8.

28. Davies DA, Yanchar NL. Appendicitis in the obese child. J Pediatr Surg 2007;42(5):857–61.

29. Gordon JE, Hughes MS, Shepherd K, et al. Obstructive sleep apnoea syndrome in morbidly obese children with tibia vara. J Bone Joint Surg Br 2006;88(1): 100–3.

30. Arkin AM, Katz JF. The effects of pressure on epiphyseal growth; the mechanism of plasticity of growing bone. J Bone Joint Surg Am 1956;38(5):1056–76.

31. Ballock RT, O'Keefe RJ. Growth and development of the skeleton. Einhorn TA ORBJ, editor. Orthopaedic basic science: foundations of clinical practice. Rosemont (IL): American Academy of Orthopaedic Surgeons; 2007. p. 115–27.

32. Villemure I, Stokes IA. Growth plate mechanics and mechanobiology. A survey of present understanding. J Biomech 2009;42(12):1793–803.

33. Grover JP, Vanderby R, Leiferman EM, et al. Mechanical behavior of the lamb growth plate in response to asymmetrical loading: a model for Blount disease. J Pediatr Orthop 2007;27(5):485–92.

34. Stokes IA, Aronsson DD, Dimock AN, et al. Endochondral growth in growth plates of three species at two anatomical locations modulated by mechanical compression and tension. J Orthop Res 2006; 24(6):1327–34.

35. Stokes IA, Clark KC, Farnum CE, et al. Alterations in the growth plate associated with growth modulation by sustained compression or distraction. Bone 2007;41(2):197–205.

36. Agamanolis DP, Weiner DS, Lloyd JK. Slipped capital femoral epiphysis: a pathological study. I. A light microscopic and histochemical study of 21 cases. J Pediatr Orthop 1985;5(1):40–6.

37. Carter JR, Leeson MC, Thompson GH, et al. Late-onset tibia vara: a histopathologic analysis. A comparative evaluation with infantile tibia vara and slipped capital femoral epiphysis. J Pediatr Orthop 1988;8(2):187–95.

38. Wenger DR, Mickelson M, Maynard JA. The evolution and histopathology of adolescent tibia vara. J Pediatr Orthop 1984;4(1):78–88.

39. Blount WP. Tibia vara, osteochondrosis deformans tibiae. Curr Pract Orthop Surg 1966;3:141–56.

40. Golding JSR, McNeil-Smith JDG. Observations on the etiology of tibia vara. J Bone Joint Surg Br 1963;45:320–5.

41. Siffert RS, Katz JF. The intra-articular deformity in osteochondrosis deformans tibiae. J Bone Joint Surg Am 1970;52(4):800–4.

42. Sabharwal S, Lee J Jr, Zhao C. Multiplanar deformity analysis of untreated Blount disease. J Pediatr Orthop 2007;27(3):260–5.

43. Hofmann A, Jones RE, Herring JA. Blount's disease after skeletal maturity. J Bone Joint Surg Am 1982;64(7):1004–9.

44. Ingvarsson T, Hagglund G, Ramgren B, et al. Long-term results after infantile Blount's disease. J Pediatr Orthop B 1998;7(3):226–9.

45. Zayer M. Osteoarthritis following Blount's disease. Int Orthop 1980;4(1):63–6.

46. Sabharwal S. Blount disease. J Bone Joint Surg Am 2009;91(7):1758–76.

47. Cook SD, Lavernia CJ, Burke SW, et al. A biomechanical analysis of the etiology of tibia vara. J Pediatr Orthop 1983;3(4):449–54.

48. Davids JR, Huskamp M, Bagley AM. A dynamic biomechanical analysis of the etiology of adolescent tibia vara. J Pediatr Orthop 1996;16(4):461–8.

49. Dietz WH Jr, Gross WL, Kirkpatrick JA Jr. Blount disease (tibia vara): another skeletal disorder associated with childhood obesity. J Pediatr 1982;101(5):735–7.

50. Gushue DL, Houck J, Lerner AL. Effects of childhood obesity on three-dimensional knee joint biomechanics during walking. J Pediatr Orthop 2005;25(6):763–8.

51. Pirpiris M, Jackson KR, Farng E, et al. Body mass index and Blount disease. J Pediatr Orthop 2006;26(5):659–63.

52. Scott AC, Kelly CH, Sullivan E. Body mass index as a prognostic factor in development of infantile Blount disease. J Pediatr Orthop 2007;27(8):921–5.

53. Bathfield CA, Beighton PH. Blount disease. A review of etiological factors in 110 patients. Clin Orthop Relat Res 1978;135:29–33.

54. Salenius P, Vankka E. The development of the tibiofemoral angle in children. J Bone Joint Surg Am 1975;57(2):259–61.

55. Henderson RC. Tibia vara: a complication of adolescent obesity. J Pediatr 1992;121(3):482–6.

56. Henderson RC, Greene WB. Etiology of late-onset tibia vara: is varus alignment a prerequisite? J Pediatr Orthop 1994;14(2):143–6.

57. Greene WB. Infantile tibia vara. J Bone Joint Surg Am 1993;75(1):130–43.

58. McIntosh AL, Hanson CM, Rathjen KE. Treatment of adolescent tibia vara with hemiepiphysiodesis: risk factors for failure. J Bone Joint Surg Am 2009;91(12):2873–9.

59. Schroerlucke S, Bertrand S, Clapp J, et al. Failure of orthofix eight-plate for the treatment of blount disease. J Pediatr Orthop 2009;29(1):57–60.

60. Stanitski DF, Dahl M, Louie K, et al. Management of late-onset tibia vara in the obese patient by using circular external fixation. J Pediatr Orthop 1997;17(5):691–4.

61. Smith SL, Beckish ML, Winters SC, et al. Treatment of late-onset tibia vara using afghan percutaneous osteotomy and orthofix external fixation. J Pediatr Orthop 2000;20(5):606–10.

62. Stevens PM, MacWilliams B, Mohr RA. Gait analysis of stapling for genu valgum. J Pediatr Orthop 2004;24(1):70–4.

63. White GR, Mencio GA. Genu valgum in children: diagnostic and therapeutic alternatives. J Am Acad Orthop Surg 1995;3(5):275–83.

64. Zhang AL, Exner GU, Wenger DR. Progressive genu valgum resulting from idiopathic lateral distal femoral physeal growth suppression in adolescents. J Pediatr Orthop 2008;28(7):752–6.

65. Manoff EM. Body mass index in patients with slipped capital femoral epiphysis. J Pediatr Orthop 2007;27(3):362–3.

66. Bhatia NN, Pirpiris M, Otsuka NY. Body mass index in patients with slipped capital femoral epiphysis. J Pediatr Orthop 2006;26(2):197–9.

67. Galbraith RT, Gelberman RH, Hajek PC, et al. Obesity and decreased femoral anteversion in adolescence. J Orthop Res 1987;5(4):523–8.

68. Mirkopulos N, Weiner DS, Askew M. The evolving slope of the proximal femoral growth plate relationship to slipped capital femoral epiphysis. J Pediatr Orthop 1988;8(3):268–73.

69. Zenios M, Ramachandran M, Axt M, et al. Posterior sloping angle of the capital femoral physis: interobserver and intraobserver reliability testing and predictor of bilaterality. J Pediatr Orthop 2007;27(7):801–4.

70. Murray AW, Wilson NI. Changing incidence of slipped capital femoral epiphysis: a relationship with obesity? J Bone Joint Surg Br 2008;90(1):92–4.

71. Benson EC, Miller M, Bosch P, et al. A new look at the incidence of slipped capital femoral epiphysis in new Mexico. J Pediatr Orthop 2008;28(5): 529–33.
72. Riad J, Bajelidze G, Gabos PG. Bilateral slipped capital femoral epiphysis: predictive factors for contralateral slip. J Pediatr Orthop 2007;27(4): 411–4.
73. Hurley JM, Betz RR, Loder RT, et al. Slipped capital femoral epiphysis. The prevalence of late contralateral slip. J Bone Joint Surg Am 1996; 78(2):226–30.
74. Kocher MS, Bishop JA, Hresko MT, et al. Prophylactic pinning of the contralateral hip after unilateral slipped capital femoral epiphysis. J Bone Joint Surg Am 2004;86(12):2658–65.
75. Barlow SE. Expert committee recommendations regarding the prevention, assessment, and treatment of child and adolescent overweight and obesity: summary report. Pediatrics 2007;120(Suppl 4): S164–92.
76. Kaufman FR, Lustig RH, Vigersky R. Patient guide to the prevention and management of pediatric obesity. J Clin Endocrinol Metab 2008;93(12):2.

Treatment of Knee Arthrosis in the Morbidly Obese Patient

Brian R. Hamlin, MD

KEYWORDS

- Total knee arthroplasty
- Unicompartmental knee arthroplasty
- Knee arthrosis • Morbid obesity

Obesity is directly linked to the development of osteoarthritis of the knee. Many of these patients will present themselves to the treating orthopedic surgeon with severe pain and disability. The morbidly obese patient may be more severely affected by their arthrosis due to its effect on their mobility and quality of life. The goal of the treating orthopedic surgeon should be to maintain a patient's mobility, improve or maintain quality of life, and provide pain relief while minimizing risk and complications of treatment.

The purpose of this article is to present the challenges that one faces when dealing with the morbidly obese patient population suffering from degenerative knee arthrosis and provide guidance for treatment options.

THE PROBLEM

The number of patients requiring total knee arthroplasty (TKA) over the next 10 to 20 years is expected to exponentially increase.[1] Many of these patients with degenerative arthritis of the knee suffer from obesity. Bourne and colleagues[2] have shown that patients with morbid obesity (body mass index [BMI] >40) have a 32 times greater likelihood than those who are normal weight (BMI <25) of requiring a total knee replacement. A linear relationship has been established with decreasing levels of glycosaminoglycans (and presumably poorer health of articular cartilage) with increasing BMI.[3] Additionally patients who are morbidly obese present

sooner for intervention, often presenting on the order of a decade younger than patients of normal weight.[4] The treating orthopedic surgeon therefore will continue to deal with this complex patient subgroup and their unique challenges. Several studies have investigated the effect of obesity on the results of total knee arthroplasty. Depending on the parameters of the study and the level of obesity variable results have been reported. Whereas many patients will be obese (BMI >30) and fare well with surgical intervention, the patient subset that truly challenges the surgeon is the morbidly obese (BMI >40). Many surgeons will choose not to offer patients of this size treatment owing to a perceived increased risk of complications as well as difficulty in performing surgery.

EVALUATION

The evaluation of a patient who is morbidly obese with knee arthrosis begins with a thorough history and physical examination. Important comorbidities to define include coronary artery disease, diabetes mellitus, and obstructive sleep apnea syndrome (OSAS). A history of venous thromboembolism (VTE), whether deep vein thrombosis or pulmonary embolus, should be noted. It is not uncommon for this patient population to suffer from chronic venous stasis (sometimes with ulcers) or lymphedema. On physical examination it is important to note the overall size and shape

The author is a consultant for Depuy/J & J but there is no conflict in relation to the article.
The Orthopaedic Program, 300 Halket Street, Magee Womens Hospital of UPMC, Pittsburgh, PA 15213, USA
E-mail address: hamlinbr@mail.magee.edu

Orthop Clin N Am 42 (2011) 107–113
doi:10.1016/j.ocl.2010.09.001

of the extremity. Patients may have a relatively normal-appearing leg and display truncal obesity, while others will have a significant amount of adiposity throughout their extremity. The patient with a normal-appearing leg does not provide as much of a surgical challenge. Range of motion should be measured paying careful attention to possible flexion contractures as well as limitations of knee flexion. Patients with a large amount of thigh and calf adiposity will have soft tissue constraints to their knee flexion. This constraint or thigh-calf impingement is important to note, as this will limit their flexion. Also if one cannot flex the knee to at least 60 degrees in the office setting (limitation due to soft tissue impingement), one will have great difficulty placing the tibial component at the time of surgery.

CONSERVATIVE TREATMENT

As in all patients with degenerative joint disease conservative treatment should be optimized before considering surgical options. The patient's obesity should be frankly discussed outlining its effect on their arthrosis and mobility and the challenges they face if and when surgical intervention is entertained. A program of weight loss should be recommended and a referral to a dietician or nutrition consultant should be offered. Often the morbidly obese patient has difficulty with a weight loss program because of knee arthrosis and its limitations on their mobility. Some of these patients may be candidates for an evaluation by a surgeon specializing in gastric surgery (gastric bypass, gastric sleeve). A study at the Mayo Clinic specifically looked into the effect of bariatric surgery before undergoing total joint arthroplasty.[5] Although the sample size was small, 20 patients underwent bariatric surgery and went on to have a successful joint replacement. The patients' BMI reduced from an average of 49 to 29 and there was an average wait of 23 months from time of bariatric surgery to joint replacement. This wait time is necessary for weight loss and to return to a noncatabolic state so they can heal their wound. If patients are taken for surgery before this time they are at risk for wound breakdown and infection from a relatively malnourished state. For a patient with end-stage arthrosis with issues with mobility and pain, this a very long time to wait for surgery.

For patients with extremely large limbs in which the soft tissue impingement will not allow access to the joint or there is such a large abdominal panniculus that the knee cannot be accessed, surgery should not be entertained. These patients must lose weight and often will require bariatric intervention. Unfortunately, bariatric surgery is not without its own risks and not all patients will be a candidate or have a successful result of this intervention. In addition, the surgery is often considered elective by insurance plans and patients will have difficulty getting coverage. The orthopedic surgeon must be the patient's advocate when this occurs and be willing to support the patient with documentation supporting the impact of their obesity on their disease as well as the benefits of bariatric surgery before joint arthroplasty.

In addition to weight loss, physical therapy for strength and flexibility, as well as instruction in a safe cardiovascular-focused exercise program, should be attempted. Aerobic programs that minimize impact loading of the joint should be encouraged. The judicious use of corticosteroid injections or viscosupplementation can help the patient to buy time and possibly work on weight loss and mobility before surgical intervention is considered. Bracing has been shown to be helpful in the treatment of knee arthritis.[6] Often the obese and particularly the morbidly obese patients have a limb that is somewhat cone shaped and therefore ill-suited for brace fitting. A lateral or medial heel wedge can be of use in the varus or valgus knee, respectively.

PREOPERATIVE OPTIMIZATION

While managing the patient's disease process conservatively, comorbidities should be optimized before surgical intervention (regardless of the type of surgery planned). Patients with coronary artery disease will require evaluation and clearance by their primary care physician or cardiologist. New cardiac disease may be discovered requiring intervention with stenting or bypass before an elective knee replacement. All patients should have a hemoglobin A1C performed to ensure their blood sugar is well controlled and to ensure they do not have unrecognized diabetes mellitus. Patients should have a value less than 8 before undergoing surgery. A recent review of a national database has shown that patients with poorly controlled or uncontrolled diabetes have higher risk of stroke, urinary tract infection, ileus, postoperative hemorrhage, transfusion, wound infection, and death.[7] Patients should be evaluated for the presence of OSAS as many undergoing total joint arthroplasty will suffer from undiagnosed OSAS at time of surgery.[8] Finally, the patient's limb should also be optimized for surgery. Chronic lymphedema should be minimized with appropriate lymphedema care, often with the use of custom compression stockings and a referral to a lymphedema nurse or clinic.

By undertaking this approach preoperatively, the risks of complications are minimized and chance of success are improved. This approach commits the patient to take an active role in the process before a major surgical procedure in which their size and comorbidities significantly effect the outcome. Surgery is not scheduled until these preoperative requirements have been met.

SURGICAL OPTIONS

Surgical options for knee arthrosis include arthroscopy, osteotomy, and arthroplasty. Knee arthroscopy with debridement and lavage of the joint is not advocated in this patient population and should be avoided. An upper tibial osteotomy for isolated medial compartment arthrosis has been shown to provide reasonable pain relief and maintenance of function for many patients[9] Unfortunately obesity has been shown to be a major predictor of failure for this intervention.[9,10] However, a corrective osteotomy may play a role in someone with isolated disease who is young and a laborer. Finally, arthroplasty may be offered for end-stage arthrosis of the knee. Unicompartmental knee arthroplasty (UKA) can be of some benefit in the patient with single-compartment involvement, but most patients will require total knee replacement.

SURGICAL EQUIPMENT

Before proceeding to surgery it is important to have proper surgical equipment and implants available. A leg holder that attaches to the operating table is very helpful (**Fig. 1**). Owing to the severe deformity of some of these knees, collateral ligament insufficiency is common as well as major bone loss or voids. Semiconstrained implants should be readily available, as well as stems, augments, and wedges. A surgical table that can hold a patient greater than 300 pounds is

necessary, as well as a bariatric bed for postoperative care.

SURGICAL PROCESS (TOTAL KNEE ARTHROPLASTY)

Two surgical assistants can be helpful for limb positioning and retraction. There is no place for minimally invasive knee surgery in this patient population. An attempt is made to exsanguinate the limb and use a standard tourniquet. If a venous tourniquet results, it is best to proceed without and only use the tourniquet for cementation of implants. Large incisions are necessary for adequate exposure and for placing retractors to protect soft tissues (**Fig. 2**). Patellar eversion will often not be possible because of the thickness of the soft tissues and, therefore, the patella should be subluxated. The sequence of the bony cuts depends on surgeon preference. There is controversy on whether a patella should be resurfaced in these patients. Obese patients have been noted to have more patellar pain whether the patella has been resurfaced[11] or not.[12] Healy and colleagues[13] found that obese patients were more likely to have loosening of their patellar component. If the decision is made to resurface the patella it may or may not be possible to evert the patella because of the large

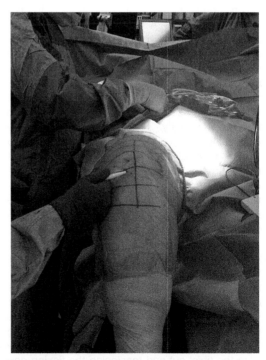

Fig. 2. Due to the large size of this patient's lower extremity, a very large surgical incision has been planned. Larger incisions are required for optimal visualization and successful arthroplasty.

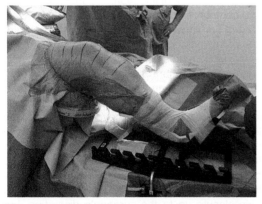

Fig. 1. A morbidly obese patient is positioned for a total knee arthroplasty. The positioner attaches to the operative table to provide additional support for this large lower extremity.

soft tissue envelope. If the patella cannot be reliably everted (and resurfacing is planned), the femoral and tibial cuts can be made first. The patella cut can then be made with the knee in extension. The tibial cut can be difficult to perform owing to an inability to flex the knee. If one makes the distal femoral cut first, it "opens" up the knee, allowing for an easier exposure for the tibial cut. The accuracy of the tibial cut, likewise, can be compromised from the large soft tissue envelope. A traditional extramedullary alignment guide can be used, but standard bony landmarks may not be easily identified. Consideration for an intramedullary alignment guide or computer-assisted navigation may be helpful and eliminate the chance of a poor tibial cut. Lozano and colleagues[14] investigated the use of an intra- versus extramedullary tibial guide as it relates to accuracy of implant position. They did not note any difference in alignment but did note a shorter operative time when using an intramedullary tibial guide in the morbidly obese patient. They concluded that the intramedullary guide allowed for a decreased operative time because of the relative ease of tibial component positioning.

Soft tissue balancing should be performed based on the experience and discretion of the surgeon. This author prefers to perform soft tissue releases in extension. Often the morbidly obese patient has severe deformity with associated flexion contracture, as well as a contracted soft tissue sleeve. A relatively aggressive soft tissue release may be necessary to achieve soft tissue balance in extension. For a severe varus deformity it may be helpful to perform a tibial reduction osteotomy, thus further relaxing the medial soft tissue sleeve. A piecrust technique is used for balancing a knee with a valgus deformity. These large releases may necessitate the use of a semiconstrained implant. It is not uncommon to have inadvertent trauma to the bone or soft tissues due to the relative force required for optimal exposure. Winiarsky and colleagues[15] reported an incidence of medial collateral ligament disruption of 8% in their study on TKA in the morbidly obese.

Patients with flexion contractures should have all posterior osteophytes removed, as well as a careful posterior capsule release. Some joint line elevation may be necessary to achieve full extension. Care should be taken to not elevate the joint line too far as it effect the patellar mechanics and may cause midflexion instability. This author prefers balancing the flexion gap with a gap-balancing technique using the tibial cut and tensioning the flexion gap with laminar spreaders. The femoral cutting block is allowed to rotate until a parallel gap is noted. This allows for a well-balanced flexion gap. The flexion gap may feel tight due to the large size of the leg.

Posterior cruciate ligament retention, sacrifice, or substitution may be used according to the surgeon's discretion. In general, substituting for the posterior cruciate ligament affords one an easier knee to balance—with the caveat of paying careful attention to not having a loose flexion gap. A spacer block technique is most helpful in assessing one's flexion and extension gaps and ensuring these are equal. Owing to the risk of flexion instability, it is this author's preference to allow the knee to be slightly tighter in flexion. During implant trialing, some tibial lift off may occur secondary to thigh-calf impingement and not necessarily because of an overly tight flexion space. In addition to there not being data on status of the cruciate, there likewise is not data on the type of tibial implant—whether it be fixed or mobile, metal backed, or all polyethylene. Often it can be difficult to place the tibial polyethylene and this author has found the rotating platform polyethylene easier to place with this group of patients.

If femoral notching occurs the femoral component should be stemmed to lessen the chance of postoperative fracture. Data does not support the association of femoral notching with a supracondylar femoral fracture.[16] Despite this, in this large patient population the author believes there is a greater likelihood of fracture if a notch occurs. There is also chance of intraoperative fracture of a femoral condyle or tibial plateau due to size of the leg and the relative force of retraction for exposure. All fractures should be stabilized with screw fixation and consideration should be given to placing stemmed implants. Appropriate instrumentation must be available for this complication and readily at hand.

There is enough data suggesting there may be an increased risk of infection,[17,18] therefore antibiotic cement (1 dose or gram of antibiotic for each 40 g of cement) is used for fixation. After completion of implantation the tourniquet is released and meticulous hemostasis is achieved. Hemostatic agents such as fibrin sealants may be helpful to minimize bleeding and lessen the chance of postoperative hematoma. Drains are placed within the joint and also superficially above the deep fascia to lessen the chance of postoperative hematoma in the dead space between the skin and capsule from the large soft tissue flaps. A meticulous closure of the deep and superficial subcutaneous tissues is necessary to decrease the dead space. Skin closure up to the surgeon's discretion, but skin staples are commonly used.

Postoperatively, patients receive standard intravenous antibiotics for 23 hours. Drains are pulled approximately 24 hours postoperatively. VTE prophylaxis involves the use of thromboembolic deterrent (TED) hose, mechanical compression, as well as chemoprophylaxis. Most studies do not indicate an increased risk for deep vein thrombosis or pulmonary embolism in the obese.[19–21] Memtsoudis and colleagues[22] did find that obesity (as well as other factors) was a predictor for an increased risk of pulmonary embolus after primary or revision hip-and-knee arthroplasty. Chemoprophylaxis is used according to the surgeons' discretion. In general, it is the author's practice to use Coumadin for a total of 6 weeks postoperatively. A Lovenox bridge is used for patients with a strong history of VTE. Some patient limbs will not allow placement of a TED hose and, therefore, are wrapped with a compression ace wrap from toes to mid-thigh. Patients are started on early mobilization including use of continuous passive motion (CPM) if the device can accommodate the size of the extremity. Aggressive knee flexion may not be beneficial for wound healing in the first 48 to 72 hours because of decreased oxygen tension at the incision site (especially with the use of large soft tissue flaps).

DIABETIC PATIENTS

All patients should have tight glucose control and monitoring. Some patients will not have true diabetes but will have elevated blood sugars due to the stress of their operative course. Data supports tight glucose control to lessen the chance of perioperative complications including wound infection.[7,23,24]

OSAS

Patients with sleep apnea should be carefully monitored, especially when receiving narcotics such as intravenous patient-controlled analgesia. Patients with known OSAS who use continuous positive airway pressure (CPAP) must be placed on CPAP postoperatively. All morbidly obese patients should be monitored for the first 24 to 48 hours with a continuous pulse oximetry and evaluated by respiratory therapist. Some patients may have undiagnosed sleep apnea at time of surgery.[8] This group is at a high risk of a serious complication. Gupta and colleagues[25] found that patients with undiagnosed OSAS were at a much greater risk for serious postoperative complications including delirium, respiratory failure, and a prolonged ICU stay.

WOUND MANAGEMENT

Wound complications can be common and must be taken seriously. Persistent drainage more than 48 to 72 hours postoperatively requires a return to the operating room for wound debridement with cultures. If there is an obvious communication or defect in the deep fascia, a deep debridement and irrigation should be performed. The polyethylene can be exchanged at this time. Antibiotics should be held until cultures have been taken. Postoperative antibiotics should be continued for 48 hours and chemoprophylaxis is halted except for aspirin. CPM is discontinued and the wound is covered with a compression dressing. If cultures are positive, antibiotics are continued for 6 weeks with an infectious disease consultant directing appropriate antibiotic therapy. Controversy exists as to the appropriateness of incision and drainage with component retention. Recent data suggests infections with methicillin-resistant *Staphylococcus aureus* (MRSA) do not fare well with this approach. Consideration should be given to explanting the components in patients with MRSA using a two-stage reimplantation.

ARTHROPLASTY

UKA, whether medial or lateral, can offer a suitable option for treatment of isolated compartmental arthrosis. Caution must be used when using this option in the morbidly obese. Data suggests obese patients may have a greater risk of loosening and, therefore, obesity is considered a relative contraindication for UKA. Berend and colleagues[26] noted a significant difference in survivorship with patients with a BMI greater than 32 using a cemented, all-polyethylene, tibial component. Some data suggest a metal-backed, mobile-bearing, medial unicompartmental design may perform well[27] in the obese, but caution should still be heeded in the morbidly obese.

TKA offers the most reproducible results for treatment of advanced arthrosis. Traditionally surgeons have been hesitant to offer the morbidly obese patient knee replacement because of concerns of failure owing to loosening, as well as the risk of complications. The assumption has been that the patients weight would lead to a higher loosening and wear rate.

Follow up data on the morbidly obese patient is mixed, but several studies hint at worsening long-term outcomes, as well as a persistent incidence of wound and infection complications. Krushell and Fingeroth[20] studied 39 TKAs in patients with a BMI greater than 40. Twenty-one percent had wound complications and two patients required revision at 5 and 10 years postoperatively. The remaining patients were pleased with their result, although their knee scores were lower than a matched cohort.

Namba and colleagues[21] found a statistically significant (P<.05) increased chance of infection in those with a BMI greater than 35. Of the patients with a BMI greater than 35, 1.1% (5 out of 422) suffered an infection versus 0.3% (4 out of 1391) with a BMI less than 35. Foran and colleagues[28] reported on comparative results of 30 patients with BMI greater or less than 30, with a follow-up for a mean of 15 years. Only 21 out of 30 (70%) of the obese group were considered successes compared with 90% (27 out of 30) of the nonobese (combining reoperation, clinical, and radiographic failure). Dewan and colleagues[29] found that BMI of less than 40 was associated with a 5.4 times likelihood of patellar radiolucencies and had more patellofemoral symptoms. They also had higher revision (7%), infection (7%), and overall complication rates (26%), but these were not significant. Foran and colleagues[30] compared 78 knees in patients with BMI greater than 30 to matched nonobese patients. Only 88% of the obese patients had a Knee Society score greater than 80 at 88 months postoperatively compared with 99% of the nonobese. Four of the obese patients required revision compared with none of the nonobese. Griffin and colleagues[31] reported 10-year results on 32 patients who were obese (BMI >30). Radiolucent lines and poorer patellar scores were more common in those with obesity, but none required revision. Jackson and colleagues[32] followed 535 consecutive patients with 153 obese and 383 nonobese (BMI <30) for an average of 9.2 years. Survivorship was not different, but the obese patients had lower improvements in their clinical Knee Society scores and worse knee flexion. Amin and colleagues[17] prospectively examined 41 consecutive patients with a BMI greater than 40 compared with a matched group with a BMI less than 30. These patients were followed for a mean of 38.5 months. The morbidly obese patients had lower Knee Society scores, a higher rate of radiolucent lines, a higher rate of complications (32% vs 0%) and poorer survivorship (73.6% vs 97.6%). Seven superficial infections and two deep infections occurred in the obese compared with none in the nonobese group.

Several investigators have noted similar problems with the wound and with infection. Dowsey and Choong[18] found that morbid obesity in those that are diabetic are at an increased risk for infection. Patients with morbid obesity were at an increased risk of 8.96 times to suffer from an infection. Malinzak and colleagues[33] found similar results looking at TKA, and patients with a BMI greater than 50 had an increased odds ratio of infection of 21.3 times.

SUMMARY

Patients with advanced arthrosis with morbid obesity present unique challenges. Conservative management should be optimized. Often patients present with advanced arthrosis that ultimately will require TKA to alleviate pain and, hopefully, allow for mobility, regaining the ability to participate in activities of daily living, and ultimately having a better quality of life. Owing to risks related to comorbidities, diligence is necessary before proceeding with surgery to lessen the chance of complications—especially infection. Surgery should only be undertaken when conservative management has failed and comorbidities optimized. The morbidly obese patient must take an active role in the management of their care especially in optimizing or preparing for surgical intervention. Although the patients can be a challenge to care for, most will benefit from surgical intervention. Patients must understand their increased risk as well as the likelihood for slightly less survivorship and satisfaction compared with patients with a normal BMI.

REFERENCES

1. Iorio R, Robb WJ, Healy WL, et al. Orthopaedic surgeon workforce and volume assessment for total hip and knee replacement in the United States: preparing for an epidemic. J Bone Joint Surg Am 2008;90(7):1598–605.
2. Bourne R, Mukhi S, Zhu N, et al. Role of obesity on the risk for total hip or knee arthroplasty. Clin Orthop Relat Res 2007;465:185–8.
3. Buchholz AL, Niesen MC, Gausden EB, et al. Metabolic activity of osteoarthritic knees correlates with BMI. Knee 2010;17(2):161–6.
4. Changulani M, Kalairajah Y, Peel T, et al. The relationship between obesity and the age at which hip and knee replacement is undertaken. J Bone Joint Surg Br 2008;90(3):360–3.
5. Parvizi J, Trousdale RT, Sarr MG. Total joint arthroplasty in patients surgically treated for morbid obesity. J Arthroplasty 2000;15(8):1003–8.
6. Kirkley A, Webster-Bogaert S, Litchfield R, et al. The effect of bracing on varus gonarthrosis. J Bone Joint Surg Am 1999;81(4):539–48.
7. Marchant MH Jr, Viens NA, Cook C, et al. The impact of glycemic control and diabetes mellitus on perioperative outcomes after total joint arthroplasty. J Bone Joint Surg Am 2009;91(7):1621–9.
8. Harrison MM, Childs A, Carson PE. Incidence of undiagnosed sleep apnea in patients scheduled

for elective total joint arthroplasty. J Arthroplasty 2003;18(8):1044–7.

9. Sprenger TR, Doerzbacher JF. Tibial osteotomy for the treatment of varus gonarthrosis. Survival and failure analysis to twenty-two years. J Bone Joint Surg Am 2003;85(3):469–74.

10. Coventry MB, Ilstrup DM, Wallrichs SL. Proximal tibial osteotomy. A critical long-term study of eighty-seven cases. J Bone Joint Surg Am 1993; 75(2):196–201.

11. Stern SH, Insall JN. Total knee arthroplasty in obese patients. J Bone Joint Surg Am 1990;72(9):1400–4.

12. Picetti GD 3rd, McGann WA, Welch RB. The patello-femoral joint after total knee arthroplasty without patellar resurfacing. J Bone Joint Surg Am 1990; 72(9):1379–82.

13. Healy WL, Wasilewski SA, Takei R, et al. Patellofe-moral complications following total knee arthro-plasty. Correlation with implant design and patient risk factors. J Arthroplasty 1995;10(2):197–201.

14. Lozano LM, Segur JM, Macule F, et al. Intramedul-lary versus extramedullary tibial cutting guide in severely obese patients undergoing total knee replacement: a randomized study of 70 patients with body mass index >35 kg/m2. Obes Surg 2008;18(12):1599–604.

15. Winiarsky R, Barth P, Lotke P. Total knee arthroplasty in morbidly obese patients. J Bone Joint Surg Am 1998;80(12):1770–4.

16. Ritter MA, Faris PM, Keating EM. Anterior femoral notching and ipsilateral supracondylar femur frac-ture in total knee arthroplasty. J Arthroplasty 1988; 3(2):185–7.

17. Amin AK, Clayton RA, Patton JT, et al. Total knee replacement in morbidly obese patients. Results of a prospective, matched study. J Bone Joint Surg Br 2006;88(10):1321–6.

18. Dowsey MM, Choong PF. Obese diabetic patients are at substantial risk for deep infection after primary TKA. Clin Orthop Relat Res 2009;467(6):1577–81.

19. Amin AK, Patton JT, Cook RE, et al. Does obesity influence the clinical outcome at five years following total knee replacement for osteoarthritis? J Bone Joint Surg Br 2006;88(3):335–40.

20. Krushell RJ, Fingeroth RJ. Primary total knee arthro-plasty in morbidly obese patients: a 5- to 14-year follow-up study. J Arthroplasty 2007;22(6 Suppl 2): 77–80.

21. Namba RS, Paxton L, Fithian DC, et al. Obesity and perioperative morbidity in total hip and total knee arthroplasty patients. J Arthroplasty 2005;20(7 Suppl 3):46–50.

22. Memtsoudis SG, Besculides MC, Gaber L, et al. Risk factors for pulmonary embolism after hip and knee arthroplasty: a population-based study. Int Orthop 2009;33(6):1739–45.

23. Dronge AS, Perkal MF, Kancir S, et al. Long-term glycemic control and postoperative infectious complications. Arch Surg 2006;141(4):375–80 [discussion: 380].

24. Kramer R, Groom R, Weldner D, et al. Glycemic control and reduction of deep sternal wound infec-tion rates: a multidisciplinary approach. Arch Surg 2008;143(5):451–6.

25. Gupta RM, Parvizi J, Hanssen AD, et al. Postopera-tive complications in patients with obstructive sleep apnea syndrome undergoing hip or knee replace-ment: a case-control study. Mayo Clin Proc 2001; 76(9):897–905.

26. Berend KR, Lombardi AV Jr, Mallory TH, et al. Early failure of minimally invasive unicompartmental knee arthroplasty is associated with obesity. Clin Orthop Relat Res 2005;440:60–6.

27. Kuipers BM, Kollen BJ, Bots PC, et al. Factors asso-ciated with reduced early survival in the Oxford phase III medial unicompartment knee replacement. Knee 2010;17(1):48–52.

28. Foran JR, Mont MA, Rajadhyaksha AD, et al. Total knee arthroplasty in obese patients: a comparison with a matched control group. J Arthroplasty 2004; 19(7):817–24.

29. Dewan A, Bertolusso R, Karastinos A, et al. Implant durability and knee function after total knee arthro-plasty in the morbidly obese patient. J Arthroplasty 2009;24(Suppl 6):89–94, e1–3.

30. Foran JR, Mont MA, Etienne G, et al. The outcome of total knee arthroplasty in obese patients. J Bone Joint Surg Am 2004;86(8):1609–15.

31. Griffin FM, Scuderi GR, Insall JN, et al. Total knee ar-throplasty in patients who were obese with 10 years followup. Clin Orthop Relat Res 1998;356:28–33.

32. Jackson MP, Sexton SA, Walter WL, et al. The impact of obesity on the mid-term outcome of cementless total knee replacement. J Bone Joint Surg Br 2009; 91(8):1044–8.

33. Malinzak RA, Ritter MA, Berend ME, et al. Morbidly obese, diabetic, younger, and unilateral joint arthro-plasty patients have elevated total joint arthroplasty infection rates. J Arthroplasty 2009;24(Suppl 6): 84–8.

Hip Disease and Hip Arthroplasty

Scott A. Wingerter, MD, PhD, Robert K. Mehrle, MD*

KEYWORDS

• Total hip arthroplasty • Hip disease • Obesity

Obesity in the United States and worldwide continues to grow. According to the Centers for Disease Control, obesity is defined as a body mass index (BMI, calculated as weight in kilograms divided by height in meters squared) greater than 30. There has been a significant increase in the prevalence of obesity in the United States over the last 20 years, with the highest percentage in Mississippi.[1] The most recent data indicate that the prevalence of obesity now exceeds 30% in most sex and age groups.[2] The percentage of obese patients undergoing total hip arthroplasty (THA) seems to be increasing at an even faster rate.[3]

Many retrospective and prospective studies have evaluated whether obesity affects outcomes and complication rates after total hip replacement, with conflicting results. However, the increase in the number of obese patients requesting THA is certain, and orthopedic surgeons performing hip arthroplasty need to be aware of potential issues to minimize complications associated with this population. This article outlines preoperative and postoperative care and describes current techniques and tools used by surgeons in obese patients to facilitate soft tissue dissection, exposure, implant placement, and closure.

PREOPERATIVE PLANNING

When considering any elective surgical intervention, detailed and thorough discussions are necessary between the patient and the surgeon. However, in the case of obese patients, preoperative counseling is even more critical before making the decision for elective THA. Obesity increases the risk of multiple medical problems, such as diabetes, hypertension, heart disease, obstructive sleep apnea, and osteoarthritis.[4] Highly obese patients undergoing THA have an increased incidence of hypertension and diabetes mellitus.[5] Each associated medical condition must be addressed before surgery; yet, in aggregate, managing multiple medical problems can be problematic and may lend themselves to increased perioperative complications. Preoperative medical clearance is mandatory to optimize the patient's medical condition before surgery. Consideration should also be made for cardiology and pulmonary evaluations if there is any concern for coronary heart disease and sleep apnea.

Another factor associated with preoperative planning for the obese patients is age at the time of surgery. The obese patient set has been shown to be in need of surgical intervention at a young age.[5–8] Furthermore, morbidly obese patients (BMI >40) have been found to be as much as 10 years younger than patients with a normal BMI at presentation for arthroplasty.[8] Maximizing nonoperative management before elective joint replacement in young patients is encouraged. It is the responsibility of the surgeon considering THA for obese and morbidly obese patients that the patients understand the implications of earlier THA, and this discussion must be held within the context of the technical challenges associated with THA in obese patients.

A common belief, or possible excuse, among the obese population is that the pain associated with arthritis prevents exercise that is necessary for weight loss. Many obese patients understand that they are significantly overweight but are

The authors have nothing to disclose.
Department of Orthopedic Surgery and Rehabilitation, University of Mississippi Medical Center, 2500 North State Street, Jackson, MS 39216, USA
* Corresponding author.
E-mail address: rmehrle@umc.edu

adamant that eliminating their pain through joint replacement will allow an increase in exercise and activity leading to weight loss; however, recent studies contradict these assertions. Several recent studies have shown that a higher percentage of obese and morbidly obese patients actually gain more than 5% of their preoperative weight after total knee arthroplasty[9] and THA.[10] Another prospective study of patients undergoing total joint replacement revealed postoperative weight gain in patients who underwent both hip and knee replacement and a significant amount of weight gain in youngpatients who underwent THA.[11]

Therefore, when evaluating an obese patient for THA, it is crucial to encourage weight loss before surgery. Recommendations should include dietary changes with possible nutrition consultation, increased physical activity, and possible bariatric surgery. Physical activity is often difficult and painful for the morbidly obese, but aquatic therapy provides an alternative that both unloads the joints and allows for increased exercise ability. When considering recommendations for bariatric surgery, no specific levels are used, but patients with a BMI of more than 45 are likely to benefit, and the option should be mentioned. Results indicate that a patient can decrease their BMI significantly and undergo successful THA within an average of 2 years between bariatric surgery and arthroplasty.[12]

Considering all the additional factors and the possibility of increased complication rates, preoperative planning and the final decision for surgery are of increased importance in the obese population. Surgery can be considered even if weight loss measures are unsuccessful, but both the surgeon and the patient need to carefully weigh all risks and benefits and proceed only after expectations are mutually understood.

SURGICAL TECHNIQUE

After the decision for surgery has been made, considerations must be made for surgical positioning, approach, and technique. As with all surgical interventions, the patient should receive the surgical technique and approach that is done best by their surgeon. The morbidly obese population has been found to require a significantly longer operating time for THA,[7] and THA in obese patients tends to result in increased intraoperative blood loss.[13,14] Soft tissue handling and exposure techniques are even more critical in obese patients because of the possibility of increased wound complications. Advantages and disadvantages exist for all surgical exposures, but the senior

author (R.K.M) has found that the posterior approach in the lateral decubitus position (**Fig. 1**) aids in improving visualization. No specific changes are necessary for the obese patient, but each step can prove more difficult. The obese patient typically needs a longer incision, more operative time devoted to exposure, and a full capsulotomy for acetabular exposure. In the lateral decubitus position, gravity aids in soft tissue retraction as the abdominal panniculus displaces anteriorly away from the operative field. The buttocks also fall away from the operative field posteriorly (see **Fig. 1**); however, the surgeon may face positioning difficulties. When placing the patient in the lateral decubitus position, it can be difficult to determine if the pelvis is positioned perpendicularly to the table because of the lack of visual and palpable landmarks. The difficulties with positioning can ultimately lead to issues with acetabular component position because of unrecognized pelvic obliquity. Therefore, more vigilance must be taken in positioning, and anatomic landmarks after acetabular exposure are necessary to obtain proper component version. The obese patient likely needs a longer incision to avoid tension on soft tissues. Although these patients may be interested in minimally invasive surgery, they are not ideal candidates for such techniques because of increased trauma to soft tissues. However, the push for minimally invasive surgery has led to better instrumentation that is compatible with obese patients, such as curved reamer handles and modified retractors.

The senior author prefers the posterior approach with complete posterior capsular and muscular repair as described by Hedley and colleagues[15] for the obese population. The technique starts with an incision over the posterior half of the greater trochanter and extends

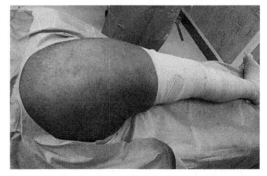

Fig. 1. An obese patient in lateral decubitus position, allowing gravity displacement of soft tissue. The abdominal panniculus is isolated from the surgical field and is not visible.

proximally and distally, with two-thirds of the incision proximal to the greater trochanter and one-third distal. A straight-line incision is created, with the leg positioned at approximately 45° of hip flexion; this positioning creates a gentle posterior curve to the incision as the leg is extended. The greater trochanter can often be difficult to palpate in obese patients. It is recommended to palpate the greater trochanter while taking the extremity through a rotational range of motion to aid in proper orientation of the incision. Palpation of the trochanter is performed during dissection through the fatty layer to ensure the correct position before reaching the fascia. The proximal extent of the exposure is critical in the obese population because the increased amount of soft tissue can prevent proper access for femoral preparation. In addition, without proper exposure, the abductor musculature can be damaged during reaming and broaching.

After the skin and subcutaneous fat dissection, the gluteus maximus muscle and iliotibial band are identified. The iliotibial band is split distally and extended proximally into a natural split in the gluteus maximus muscle. Allowing for an appropriate split in the muscle aids in minimizing the soft tissue trauma that can occur with a forced separation. A Charnley retractor is then placed to maintain exposure. In the obese population, the deeper blades for each side of the Charnley retractor need to be available and used (**Fig. 2**). Richardson retractors are then used to sequentially retract the gluteus maximus muscle anteriorly, followed by identification and retraction of the posterior border of the gluteus medius muscle to identify the interval between the gluteus medius and gluteus minimus muscles. The piriformis muscle tendon is identified along the interval with the gluteus minimus muscle.

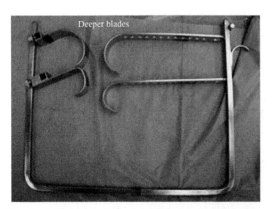

Fig. 2. A Charnley self-retaining retractor. Note the deeper blades that are necessary for retraction of soft tissues in obese and morbidly obese patients.

At this stage, a long Bovie electrocautery tip is used to ease deep dissection. The piriformis is clamped and released from its insertion on the piriformis fossa of the femur. This procedure allows access to the posterior border of the gluteus minimus, which is then dissected and elevated, off the capsule. The small Richardson retractor is then placed deep to the gluteus minimus between the muscle and the capsule. The capsule is then incised in line with the superior border of the piriformis. The capsule and short external rotator muscles are dissected off the posterior femur as one triangular flap, keeping this as long as possible for future repair.

An anterior superior capsulotomy is performed with a large curved scissors before dislocation of the femoral head. The femoral neck osteotomy is then performed at a level based on preoperative templating and intraoperative measurement from the proximal aspect of the lesser trochanter to a point representing the proposed center of the prosthetic head. The senior author has found that a full capsulotomy in this patient population is necessary to obtain proper acetabular exposure.

The second Charnley-type self-retaining retractor (**Fig. 3**) is then placed with one side firmly seated in the capsule and the other in the posterior aspect of the greater trochanter. The seating in the capsule is facilitated by a making a 2-mm hole in the capsule with Bovie electrocautery before placement. The prong can then be placed securely in this opening in the capsule. A third Charnley-type self-retaining retractor is then placed with the 4-prong side in the gluteus minimus muscle and capsule and the 2-prong side in the inferior capsule (see **Fig. 3**). The Charnley-type retractors provide long handles and hinges between blades and arms to allow proper positioning even in deep wounds (DePuy Orthopaedics, Inc, Warsaw, IN, USA). The final retractor used is the anterior retractor, which allows further anterior translation of the femur. With proper placement of all retractors, sufficient visualization of the acetabulum can be achieved even in the obese population (**Fig. 4**).

The labrum is removed from the edge of the acetabulum, and the fatty tissue is excised from the cotyloid fossa. Proper component positioning is difficult in the morbidly obese patient because of the loss of palpable and visual landmarks and tissue interference while reaming. A curved reamer handle is helpful in avoiding this interference and preventing soft tissue damage in the distal aspect of the wound in obese patients. The reaming begins with medialization to the true acetabular floor, followed by appropriate peripheral reaming. The reaming also progresses proximally to the

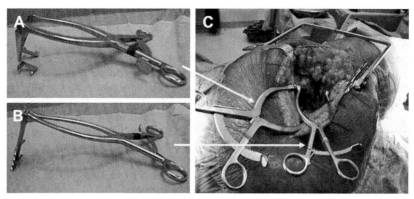

Fig. 3. (A–C) Charnley-type self-retaining retractors.

level of the teardrop so that the inferior border of the reamer and subsequently the implant is at this level. Curved handles for both the trial and final acetabular implants (**Fig. 5**) are also used to aid in prevention of vertical implant placement. Additional fixation with screws is strongly considered if a secure initial fit is not obtained.

Attention is then turned to the femur, and a curved retractor is placed under the femoral neck. A bent Hohman retractor is then placed deep to the gluteus minimus muscle to protect the abductors during femoral preparation. During trialing, the distance from the lesser trochanter to the new femoral head is measured and matched with the measurement obtained during preoperative templating. All possible soft tissue and bony impingement structures, such as redundant capsule and osteophytes, are removed before reduction and trialing. For the obese population, a stable range of motion with internal rotation to

75° to 90° with the hip at 45° flexion is satisfactory; because the soft tissue impingement is often encountered in the abdomen, range-of-motion stability is difficult to test at the desired 90° hip flexion.

No changes are required regarding the use of cemented or press-fit acetabular cups and the type of femoral stems for normal-weight or obese patients. With the final implants in place, the posterior capsule is repaired to the posterior aspect of the femur using bone tunnels and nonabsorbable suture. The remainder of the closure is routine, with the exception of an additional fat-layer closure with absorbable braided suture to decrease dead space. A drain is not routinely used for wound management. For skin closure, absorbable subcuticular stitch or skin staples are used, with an increased likelihood of using skin staples in the morbidly obese patients. If the patient is noted to have excess fluid, tension

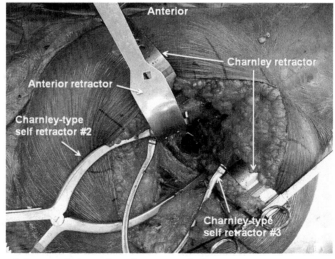

Fig. 4. Final exposure of the acetabulum after placement of all retractors.

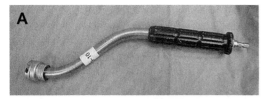

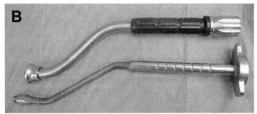

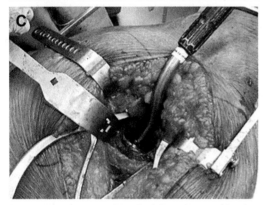

Fig. 5. Curved reamer handle (*A*) and curved implant holders (*B*). Note how the curve to the handle allows for correct orientation of the acetabular component, while limiting the interference from the excessive soft tissue sleeve (*C*).

on the closure, or a history of prolonged drainage with any previous surgery, the use of an incisional wound vacuum-assisted closure (VAC) device can be considered.

POSTOPERATIVE CARE

Patients should remain in the hospital until safe for discharge from a physical therapy standpoint and there is no drainage from the incision site. These factors may be part of the reason for conflicting evidence regarding length of stay for the obese population undergoing total hip replacement. A retrospective review has indicated a significant increase in length of stay for both overweight and obese groups,[16] whereas another large study of both total hip and total knee replacement patients showed no significant difference in length of stay between patients with BMI greater and lesser than 35.[5] However, a wide variation exists both internationally and within the United States

in the typical length of stay after THA, with averages ranging from 2 to 10 days.[5,16]

The postoperative plan of care is not significantly changed for the obese patient undergoing THA. When a posterior surgical exposure approach is used, patients must be instructed on posterior hip precautions during physical therapy, but they are allowed to begin full weight bearing as tolerated on the first postoperative day. The typical progression includes ambulation, initially with a walker, followed by advancement to a cane, and eventually to no assistive devices as per physical therapy instruction and recommendations. Overall, no changes are made to the physical therapy plan for the obese patient population.

Prolonged wound drainage is a concern in the obese population undergoing any surgical procedure. Morbid obesity has been shown to be a significant independent risk factor for prolonged wound drainage after THA.[17] Prolonged wound drainage can lead to other complications, primarily wound infection, and increased length of hospital stay. When wound drainage is noted in the early postoperative period, measures such as a compressive spica dressing should be used. A hip spica dressing is placed by wrapping 6-inch (Ace wraps 3M, St Paul, MN, USA) in a figure-of-eight pattern around the proximal thigh and waist, with the crossing point directly over the wound to provide compression at the site of the incision. Although effective for stopping persistent wound drainage, the spica dressing can be onerous with obese and morbidly obese patients. If persistent drainage is present 5 to 7 days after surgery, strong consideration should be made for a return to the operating room for irrigation and debridement because of the increased risk of infection. The use of an incisional VAC device should again be considered at this return procedure.

OUTCOMES AND COMPLICATIONS

Overall, the literature has been positive in terms of outcomes for the obese population. Many studies have shown no significant increase in complications,[7,13,14,18,19] and patient satisfaction seems to be comparable to the general population undergoing THA.[6,20] Postoperative evaluation of range of motion and Harris Hip Scores identified significantly lower results for the obese group, but the overall patient satisfaction was comparable.[6] Outcome measures often need to be evaluated on a change-in-score basis as opposed to absolute numbers for obesity studies because of the significantly lower preoperative scores and function within the obese group. Preoperative range of motion and activity level, for example, are likely much less for an obese patient, but they may still show significant improvement after surgery. Obesity has been associated with some functional limitations, such as ascending or descending stairs, compared with nonobese patients after THA, but no difference was noted with regard to patient satisfaction, decision to repeat surgery, and outcome scores.[21]

The most concerning complications are dislocation and revision rates, wound dehiscence or prolonged drainage and late infections, and systemic complications such as deep vein thrombosis or pulmonary embolism. There is conflicting evidence related to systemic complications. One study found no difference in deep vein thrombosis or pulmonary embolism rates at 5 years,[7] but another study has identified a 58% increased risk of systemic complications, such as venous thromboembolism and cardiac events, in patients with a high BMI.[16]

As with all THA literature, large variations exist in dislocation rates relative to obesity. Smaller studies have shown no significant association between high BMI and dislocation risk.[22–24] Among larger studies, dislocation rates range from less than 1%, with no significant differences based on obesity,[5] to as high as 4% in the obese population, with a significant increase compared with normal-weight patients.[25] A multicenter study comparing patients who were nonobese (BMI <30), obese (BMI, 30–40), and morbidly obese (BMI >40) found no significant difference in dislocation rates, possibly because of smaller numbers in the morbidly obese group, but there was an increased incidence of dislocation with increasing BMI.[7] Although the documented results raise some question regarding an association between obesity and dislocation rate, the possibility of increased risk indicates that surgical technique and proper implant positioning are even more crucial considerations in the obese population.

Perhaps the most significant area of concern remains wound problems and infection. Combined studies evaluating total hip and total knee replacements revealed a significantly higher rate of infection and an increased odds ratio for infection in patients with a BMI greater than 50. However, further evaluation identified that the increase in infection rates was associated with TKA and not with THA,[26] which corroborated smaller earlier studies that found no wound or infection issues in the obese patients after THA.[13] Another prospective study found a 4.2-times higher risk for infection in obese patients who underwent THA, but the increase was not found to be statistically significant. The increased risk was observed in the highly obese group (BMI>35), which included only 14% of the patients in the study.[5]

SUMMARY

Obesity is a problem that will affect the future of arthroplasty practices, and a thorough understanding of the implications is necessary for all orthopedic surgeons. The evidence remains conflicting regarding complications, such as wound drainage, infection, and dislocation, but is encouraging in that the obese population can benefit from total joint replacement after complete preoperative optimization. Detailed discussions and attempts at weight loss should be implemented and variations in surgical technique and instruments should be used to maximize outcome potential.

REFERENCES

1. Centers for Disease Control and Prevention. U.S. obesity trends: trends by state 1985–2009. Available at: http://www.cdc.gov/obesity/data/trends.html. Last updated July 27, 2010. Accessed August 22, 2010.
2. Flegal KM, Carroll MD, Ogden CL, et al. Prevalence and trends in obesity among US adults, 1999-2008. JAMA 2010;303(3):235–41.
3. Fehring TK, Odum SM, Griffin WL, et al. The obesity epidemic: its effect on total joint arthroplasty. J Arthroplasty 2007;22(6):71–6.
4. Malnick SD, Knobler H. The medical complications of obesity. QJM 2006;99(9):565–79.
5. Namba RS, Paxton L, Fithian DC, et al. Obesity and perioperative morbidity in total hip and total knee arthroplasty patients. J Arthroplasty 2005;20(7): 46–50.
6. Jackson MP, Sexton SA, Yeung E, et al. The effect of obesity on the mid-term survival and clinical outcome of cementless total hip replacement. J Bone Joint Surg Br 2009;91:1296–300.
7. Andrew JG, Palan J, Kurup HV, et al. Obesity in total hip replacement. J Bone Joint Surg Br 2008;90: 424–9.
8. Changulani M, Kalairajah Y, Peel T, et al. The relationship between obesity and the age at which hip and knee replacement is undertaken. J Bone Joint Surg Br 2008;90:360–3.
9. Dowsey MM, Liew D, Stoney JD, et al. The impact of pre-operative obesity on weight change and outcome in total knee replacement: a prospective study of 529 patients. J Bone Joint Surg Br 2010; 92(4):513–20.
10. Dowsey MM, Liew D, Stoney JD, et al. The impact of obesity on weight change and outcomes at

12 months in patients undergoing total hip arthroplasty. Med J Aust 2010;193(1):17–21.

11. Heisel C, Silva M, dela Rosa MA, et al. The effects of lower-extremity total joint replacement for arthritis on obesity. Orthopedics 2005;28(2):157–9.

12. Parvizi J, Trousdale RT, Sarr MG. Total joint arthroplasty in patients surgically treated for morbid obesity. J Arthroplasty 2000;15(8):1003–8.

13. Soballe K, Christensen F, Luxhoj T. Hip replacement in obese patients. Acta Orthop Scand 1987;58(3):223–5.

14. Lehman DE, Capello WN, Feinberg JR. Total hip arthroplasty without cement in obese patients: a minimum two-year clinical and radiographic follow-up study. J Bone Joint Surg Am 1994;76:854–62.

15. Hedley AK, Hendren DH, Mead LP. A posterior approach to the hip joint with complete posterior capsular and muscular repair. J Arthroplasty 1990;5(Suppl):S57–66.

16. Sadr Azodi O, Bellocco R, Eriksson K, et al. The impact of tobacco use and body mass index on the length of stay in hospital and the risk of postoperative complications among patients undergoing total hip replacement. J Bone Joint Surg Br 2006;88:1316–20.

17. Patel VP, Walsh M, Sehgal B, et al. Factors associated with prolonged wound drainage after primary total hip and knee arthroplasty. J Bone Joint Surg Am 2007;89:33–8.

18. Haverkamp D, de Man HR, de Jong PT, et al. Is the long-term outcome of cemented THA jeopardized by patients being overweight? Clin Orthop Relat Res 2008;466:1162–8.

19. Jiganti JJ, Goldstein WM, Williams CS. A comparison of the perioperative morbidity in total joint arthroplasty in the obese and nonobese patient. Clin Orthop Relat Res 1993;289:175–9.

20. Yeung E, Jackson M, Sexton S, et al. The effect of obesity on the outcome of hip and knee arthroplasty. Int Orthop 2010. [Epub ahead of print].

21. Stickles B, Phillips L, Brox WT, et al. Defining the relationship between obesity and total joint arthroplasty. Obes Res 2001;9(3):219–23.

22. Woolson ST, Rahimtoola ZO. Risk factors for dislocation during the first three months after primary total hip replacement. J Arthroplasty 1999;14:662–8.

23. Khatod M, Barber T, Paxton E, et al. An analysis of risk of hip dislocation with a contemporary total joint registry. Clin Orthop 2006;447:19–23.

24. McLaughlin JR, Lee KR. The outcome of total hip replacement in obese and non-obese patients at 10 to 18-years. J Bone Joint Surg Br 2006;88:1286–92.

25. Sadr Azodi O, Adami J, Lindstrom D, et al. High body mass index is associated with increased risk of implant dislocation following primary total hip replacement: 2,106 patients followed for up to 8 years. Acta Orthop 2008;79(1):141–7.

26. Malinzak RA, Ritter MA, Berend ME, et al. Morbidly obese, diabetic, younger, and unilateral joint arthroplasty patients have elevated total joint arthroplasty infection rates. J Arthroplasty 2009;24(6):84–8.

Financial Implications of Obesity

George V. Russell, MD[a,*], Christine W. Pierce, MD[a],
Loren Nunley, BA[b]

KEYWORDS

• Obesity • Societal costs • Orthopedics • Reimbursement

SOCIETAL COSTS

"Obesity outranks both smoking and drinking in its deleterious effects on health and health costs."[1] Excessive alcohol consumption and smoking have been recognized as considerable public health issues, particularly because these behaviors lead to chronic medical diseases that command considerable personal and societal resources to treat. In evaluating 1998 data from Healthcare for Communities, Sturm[1] reported that obesity was associated with a 36% increase in inpatient and outpatient spending compared with a 21% increase in inpatient and outpatient spending for smokers and excessive drinkers.[1] Although this is startling, it becomes more so when considering the greater number of obese people than smokers and excessive drinkers, the growing epidemic of obesity, and the many chronic conditions associated with obesity.

Several associated comorbidities have been linked to obesity: coronary artery disease, hypertension, type 2 diabetes mellitus, end-stage renal disease, cholecystitis, obstructive sleep apnea, breast cancer, endometrial cancer, renal cell cancer, colorectal cancer, low back pain, and arthritis. In aggregate, the direct costs for providing care for these obesity-related conditions in 1999 dollars were $331.4 billion and that portion attributed to obesity was $102.2 billion.[2] As the number of obese people increases, so do the medical costs. In 2008 dollars, costs to treat obesity totaled approximately $147 billion.[3]

Costs are commonly grouped into direct and indirect costs. Direct costs are defined as those costs associated with the diagnosis and treatment of diseases as well as treatment of the disease itself. Direct costs include costs, such as hospital and nursing home care, physician visits, and medications.[4,5] Indirect costs are the value of lost output because of cessation or reduction of productivity caused by morbidity and mortality. Examples of indirect costs are lost wages caused by absenteeism or loss of future earnings caused by premature death.[4,5] Wolf and Colditz[5] estimated the direct costs of obesity in 1998 using data from the 1988 and 1944 National Health Interview Survey and concluded that the direct costs associated with obesity were $99.2 billion and approximately $51.64 billion of that was attributed to direct medical costs. The cost of lost productivity (indirect costs) associated with obesity was $3.9 billion and reflected 39.2 million days of lost work.[5] Finkelstein and colleagues,[6] using a different data set, estimated that obesity-attributable spending accounted for 9.1% of total US medical expenditures in 1998 for a total of $78.5 billion, which equals $92.6 in 2002 dollars.[6]

The personal costs of obesity do not receive as much attention as the economic costs; however, personal costs of obesity are considerable. Discrimination against obese people is commonplace in society at large and in the health care arena.[7] A perception of lower class citizenship, whether or not real, may have profound implications on the lives of the obese. Personal costs of obesity are not commonly quantified, but it has been shown that obese subjects earn less than their lean counterparts after corrections are made for intellectual ability and social background.[4] Poor physical function may also limit earning potential. As patients are required to pay

[a] Department of Orthopaedic Surgery, University of Mississippi Medical Center, 2500 North State Street, Jackson, MS 39216, USA
[b] Howard University College of Medicine, 4201 Cathedral Avenue, NW # 218, Washington, DC 20016, USA
* Corresponding author.
E-mail address: gvrussell@umc.edu

Orthop Clin N Am 42 (2011) 123–127
doi:10.1016/j.ocl.2010.09.003

more for their health care, costs typically associated with direct costs may be attributed to personal costs, such as increased payments for insurance or higher costs for medicines.[4]

WORKPLACE COSTS

Several investigators have discussed the economic impact of obesity on the workplace. In 2000, private business expense for health services consumed 40% of pretax profits and 58% of after tax profits.[8] Thompson and colleagues[9] estimated the actual dollars spent by US businesses on health care for obese employees at $12.7 billion, including $2.6 billion for mild obesity (body mass index [BMI] 25–28.9) and $10.1 billion due to all others with a BMI greater than or equal to 29.[9]

Direct costs to employers have been explored. Burton and colleagues[10] evaluated the increased costs associated with BMI in a workplace of approximately 6500 employees. They reported the mean health care costs for employees with a BMI greater than or equal to 28 (approximate) were $6882 in comparison with $4496 for employees with BMI less than 28 (approximate).[10] In another study by Finkelstein and colleagues,[11] using the National Health Interview Survey and the Medical Expenditure Panel Survey (MEPS), the investigators found that overweight and obesity costs ranged from $175 per year for overweight male employees to $2485 for grade II obese (BMI 35.0–39.9) female employees. The investigators further estimated that the costs of obesity (excluding overweight) at a firm with 1000 employees would be $285,000 per year.[11] In looking at total costs, obesity-attributable business expenditures on paid sick leave, life insurance, and disability insurance amounted to $2.4 billion, $1.8 billion, and $800 million, respectively, in 1994.[9]

Indirect costs are also considerable for the workplace, particularly evident in employee absenteeism. Tucker and Friedman[12] evaluated more than 10,000 employees who participated in an ongoing wellness screening program. The obese employees were 1.74 and 1.61 times more likely to experience high (7 or more absences due to illness within 6 months) and moderate (3–6 absences due to illness within 6 months) levels of absenteeism, respectively, than were lean individuals.[12] Burton and colleagues[10] found that employees with a BMI greater than or equal to 27.8 for men and BMI greater than or equal to 27.3 for women experienced twice as many sick days as lean employees. They were further able to document a direct correlation between increasing BMI and absenteeism.[10] Using 1994 data, Wolf and Colditz[5] estimated the cost of lost productivity attributed to employees with a BMI greater than 30 was $3.9 billion, which reflected 39.2 million days of lost work.[5]

Despite the high cost of absenteeism to businesses, the true indirect costs must also include increased disability rates, higher employee injury rates, and presenteeism—all of which push indirect costs even higher. Presenteeism is defined as lower work output. Obese employees place a presenteeism burden on businesses due to several causes, such as physical inability to perform tasks efficiently or increased fatigue. Wolf and Colditz[5] estimated restricted activity workdays at 181,540,000 for employees with a BMI greater than or equal to 25 compared with 239 million restricted activity workdays in employees with BMI greater than or equal to 30.

WHO PAYS?

Although the discussion of health care costs attributable to obesity is stimulating, the logical next question is, Who pays for health care for obese patients? Private insurance companies do not externally publish data on this subject or at least the authors were unable to secure such data. The senior author even asked a local medical director of a large insurance company and was told the data could not be made available. Estimates have been done to determine how much is paid and who pays for obesity-related health care issues. Using data from the Bureau of Labor Statistics, Thompson and colleagues[9] estimated that of the $12.7 billion obesity-related costs to US businesses, $7.7 billion was paid out for health insurance expenditures.[9] In 1998, national medical spending for obesity, excluding overweight, was $26.8 billion, using MEPS data, or $47.5 billion, using National Health Accounts (NHA) data. Despite the different methodologies, both the MEPS and NHA estimates revealed that the public sector was responsible for financing nearly half of medical spending for obesity-attributable diseases.[11] In a recent follow-up study, Finkelstein and colleagues[13] found that the increased prevalence of obesity was responsible for almost $40 billion of increased medical spending through 2006, including $7 billion in Medicare prescription drug costs. They estimated that the medical costs of obesity could have risen to $147 billion per year by 2008.[13]

IMPLICATIONS FOR ORTHOPEDICS

Obesity has a significant impact on musculoskeletal disease. Arguably, those orthopedic surgeons who treat patients with arthritis and those patients who have been involved in trauma experience the biggest burden for care of the obese in orthopedics. Specifically, 16% of underweight/normal weight people report doctor-diagnosed arthritis compared with 21.7% of overweight and 30.6% of obese people.[14] Yet the total number of people diagnosed with arthritis by 2030 is expected to climb to an estimated 67 million Americans.[15] It can be surmised from the data that the increasing obesity epidemic, combined with the increasing number of patients with arthritis, will create a significant burden on the services of orthopedic surgeons who perform hip and knee arthroplasty procedures. A similar trend is seen in the trauma setting. The incidence of blunt trauma continues to increase. As the population gets larger, it can be expected that more obese traumatized patients will be seen who require operative care.

Caring for obese patients demands more effort than caring for nonobese patients. Many obese patients suffer from deconditioning and must be counseled and encouraged to participate in exercise to improve health. Diet and nutrition are also discussions that frequently occur and require more provider time. Additionally, if an obese patient is contemplating surgery, more time is spent by the provider in discussing comorbid conditions and arranging for preoperative evaluations by primary care physicians and other specialists. Even more time is then spent by the provider and/or the staff to ensure that recommendations are received and implemented before surgery. Of the estimated $23 billion cost of arthritis in 1999, $7.4 billion was attributed to obesity-related causes of obesity (American Obesity Society),[2] and, although the trauma setting is different, more time is spent by all providers resuscitating obese traumatized patients.

Operative care of obese patients requires more time and is more difficult. The authors of the previous articles have done an excellent job in pulling together the literature and combining it with their personal experiences to explain the difficulties in operatively treating obese patients. To offset the increased time and difficulty in operatively treating obese patients, a 22-modifier to the Current Procedural Terminology (CPT) code may be appended. A CPT code modifier "provides the means by which the reporting physician can indicate that a service or procedure that has been performed has been altered by some specific circumstance but not changed in its definition or code." The 22-modifier is one such modifier that may be used "when the service(s) provided is greater than that usually required for the listed procedure."[16] The purpose of attaching the 22-modifier is to provide additional reimbursement to the surgeon for the increased complexity of the

case under a variety of circumstances. The upcharge for a 22-modifier is different for each provider, but most payers add a percentage to the standard charge to account for a 22-modifier.

An astute observer can immediately see several problems. There are no clearly defined conditions under which a 22-modifier may be appended—they are left to the discretion of the surgeon. Therefore, what may be routine for one surgeon may be extra difficult for another, which may lead to inconsistent use of 22-modifiers. Without clearly defined criteria for using a 22-modifier, the payer has no absolute obligation to pay the upcharge. Surgeons may then avoid treating obese patients because their efforts are not adequately reimbursed.

Not much has been written about the usefulness of the 22-modifier to affect increased payments for operating on obese patients. Christensen and Jacobs,[17] in a 2009 poster presentation at the American Academy of Orthopaedic Surgeons annual meeting, observed that the 22-modifier was not adequately reimbursed in their practice. Specifically, for 93 morbidly obese patients, in cases where Medicare was the primary payer, they were reimbursed only three times for the 22-modifier.[17] Fehring and colleagues[18] applied the 22-modifier to 60 obese patients undergoing arthroplasty procedures, and in only one patient was an additional payment received from Medicare.[18] Preliminary data from ongoing research at the authors' institution corroborate these findings in a trauma model.

Related studies in other disciplines have been published regarding the usefulness of the 22-modifer to affect reimbursement. In the urology literature, Lotan and colleagues[19] sought to determine if urologists were fairly compensated for difficult procedures with the use of the 22-modifier. They analyzed their use of the 22-modifier for any surgery for a 21-month period and excluded any charity cases. They found increased reimbursement in 31% of cases with a 22-modifier, nearly equal reimbursement in 36%, and reimbursement at less than contract level in 33% of their cases. They concluded that the 22-modifier did not provide consistent additional reimbursement for more complex surgery.[19]

IMPLICATIONS FOR HOSPITALS

Hospitals also bear additional costs to care for obese patients. Obese patients have longer hospital stays and have more complications that add to the costs borne by hospitals. Hospitals are paid differently from surgeons, however, which may mitigate the additional costs. Huber and colleagues[20] highlighted the difference in a study related to vascular surgery. The investigators did not study the usefulness of the 22-modifier but studied reimbursement for procedures deemed tertiary care (thoracoabdominal aneurysms, infected aortic grafts, and chronic mesenteric ischemia) compared with those considered elective primary care (carotid endarterectomy and infrarenal aortic reconstruction). There was a dramatic difference in surgeon work effort reflected by operating room time and total care time for the tertiary procedures compared with the primary procedures, whereas there was a significantly less estimated reimbursement per surgeon work effort for the tertiary procedures. They found that providing care for these more complex procedures was still currently profitable to the academic hospital but was associated with marginal losses to the department of surgery.[20]

As highlighted by Huber and colleagues, hospitals are reimbursed differently from surgeons and perhaps, it could be argued, more favorably. In general terms, there are four classes of payers: self-pay, Medicare/private insurance, Medicaid, and charity. Self-pay models, where patients pay fee for service, are exceptions to the observation of preferential payment to hospitals over providers. In the self-pay model, the hospital and the providers are reimbursed at market rates.

Medicaid, at least in the authors' state, reimburses physicians based on CPT codes, although the rate of payment is far below market price. In an ongoing study at the authors' institution looking at 22-modifier payments, Medicaid did not increase payment for any patient. Hospitals are reimbursed on a per diem basis. It is difficult to know if this is profitable for a hospital because profit or loss depends on the per diem cost for each particular hospital. The hospitals that can provide per diem care to patients for less than Medicaid per diem rates stand to make a profit. Hospitals unable to care for patients at or below the Medicaid per diem reimbursement rate will have a loss. If a hospital is designated as a Disproportionate Share Hospital (DSH), however, then the hospital is may receive additional federal money to care for patients, whereas providers are not eligible for such additional payments.

Medicaid DSH payments provide financial assistance to hospitals that serve many low-income patients. Medicaid DSH payments are the largest source of federal funding for uncompensated hospital care.[21] "Eligible hospitals are referred to as DSH hospitals. States receive an annual DSH allotment to cover the costs of DSH hospitals that provide care to low-income patients that are not paid by other payers, such as Medicare, Medicaid, the Children's Health Insurance

Program, or other health insurance. This annual allotment is calculated by law and includes requirements to ensure that the DSH payments to individual DSH hospitals are not higher than these actual uncompensated costs."[22] "State Medicaid DSH programs and payments vary considerably."[23] States have discretion to determine which hospitals get DSH payments and how much each of them receives.[21] After the increase authorized by the American Recovery and Reinvestment Act of 2009, it is estimated that the total federal Medicaid DSH allotments available to states would increase by $269 million to approximately $11.34 billion.[22]

Hospitals may also qualify for Medicare DSH funds. The primary method for a hospital to qualify for Medicare DSH is based on the hospital's DSH patient percentage (DPP), which is defined as the sum of

- The percentage of the hospital's total Medicare patient days attributable to Medicare patients who also are federal Supplemental Security Income beneficiaries, and
- The percentage of the hospital's total patient days attributable to Medicaid beneficiaries (excluding Medicare beneficiaries)
- Hospitals whose DPP exceeds 15% are eligible for a DSH payment adjustment.

Large urban hospitals that can demonstrate that more than 30% of their total net inpatient care revenues come from state and local governments for indigent care (other than Medicare or Medicaid) also qualify for a Medicare DSH payment adjustment.[21]

A disconnect is readily evident between hospital reimbursement and provider reimbursement for complex care, in which treatment of obese patients may be classified. Huber and colleagues[20] showed in their Medicare patient subset that the net income to the hospital was greater for primary procedures and lower for tertiary procedures. Two of the three tertiary procedures demonstrated net losses; yet, reimbursement for all five evaluated procedures exceeded the direct variable costs. In evaluating physician compensation, the reimbursement per relative value unit (RVU) fell below the average estimated clinical cost per RVU, thereby creating a net loss to the providers for each of the five procedures. Fehring and colleagues[18] reported that from 1990 to 2005 in an obese Medicare patient population, their hospital showed an increase of 2.8% reimbursement in inflation adjusted dollars, whereas the physicians experienced a 59% decrease reimbursement for total knee arthroplasties and a 64% decrease for total hip arthroplasties in inflation adjusted dollars. And, as discussed previously, their attempts to capture increased reimbursement from Medicare using a 22-modifier was successful in only 1 of 60 patients. No mention was made of DSH payments to the hospital in either article.

In dealing with charity care patients, neither the hospital nor the provider theoretically collects reimbursement for services provided. Providers that work in areas with a large indigent population, however, may negotiate salary offsets or other opportunities to help defray the costs of providing indigent care. Hospitals may use a DSH designation to receive additional funding. Other opportunities may also be available for hospitals to negotiate funding opportunities, such as a state-funded program to care for indigent traumatized patients.

SUMMARY

The obesity epidemic continues to grow. As the number of obese people increases, it is logical to expect an increasing number of obese patients and increasing costs to care for these patients. Orthopedic surgeons will see many of these patients who need treatment for injuries and chronic conditions. As the authors in this issue discuss, care of obese patients requires more work and time in providing nonoperative and operative care. To date, no system has been proposed to handle reimbursement disparities, particularly for providers. As the Patient Protection and Affordable Care Act moves forward, DSH payments to hospitals are scheduled to be phased out. The model for health care will change, and along with it should be all parties coming together to address inequalities and inequities in our care for obese and morbidly patients.

REFERENCES

1. Sturm R. The effects of obesity, smoking, and drinking on medical problems and costs. Health Aff (Millwood) 2002;21(2):245–53.
2. Costs of obesity. edited; American Obesity Association. Available at: http://aoaweb.obesity.org/treatment/cost.shtml. Accessed October 4, 2010.
3. Vital Statistics. edited; Centers for Disease Control and Prevention. Available at: http://www.cdc.gov/vitalsigns/AdultObesity/index.html. Accessed October 4, 2010.
4. Seidell JC. Societal and personal costs of obesity. Exp Clin Endocrinol Diabetes 1998;106(Suppl 2):7–9.
5. Wolf AM, Colditz GA. Current estimates of the economic cost of obesity in the United States. Obes Res 1998;6(2):97–106.
6. Finkelstein EA, Fiebelkorn IC, Wang G. National medical spending attributable to overweight and obesity: how much, and who's paying? Health Aff Web Exclusives; 2003. p. 219, 26.
7. Porter SE. Office and hospital special needs for the treatment of the obese patient. Philadelphia: OCNA; 2010.
8. Cowan CA, McDonnell PA, Levit KR, et al. Burden of health care costs: businesses, households, and governments, 1987–2000. Health Care Financ Rev 2002;23(3):131–59.
9. Thompson D, Edelsberg J, Kinsey KL, et al. Estimated economic costs of obesity to U.S. business. Am J Health Promot 1998;13(2):120–7.
10. Burton WN, Chen CY, Schultz AB, et al. The economic costs associated with body mass index in a workplace. J Occup Environ Med 1998;40(9):786–92.
11. Finkelstein E, Fiebelkorn C, Wang G. The costs of obesity among full-time employees. Am J Health Promot 2005;20(1):45–51.
12. Tucker LA, Friedman GM. Obesity and absenteeism: an epidemiologic study of 10,825 employed adults. Am J Health Promot 1998;12(3):202–7.
13. Finkelstein EA, Trogdon JG, Cohen JW, et al. Annual medical spending attributable to obesity: payer-and service-specific estimates. Health Aff (Millwood) 2009;28(5):w822–31.
14. Arthritis—data statistics. edited; Centers for Disease Control and Prevention. Available at: http://www.cdc.gov/arthritis/data_statistics/arthritis_related_stats.htm. Accessed October 4, 2010.
15. Hootman JM, Helmick CG. Projections of US prevalence of arthritis and associated activity limitations. Arthritis Rheum 2006;54(1):226–9.
16. Abraham M, Beebe M, Dalton J, editors. Current procedural terminology. Chicago: American Medical Association; 2010. p. 529.
17. Christensen C, Jacobs C. In: Poster Presentation of the 2009. Annual Meeting of American Academy of Orthopaedic Surgeons. Las Vegas; 2009. p. 234.
18. Fehring TK, Odum SM, Griffin WL, et al. The obesity epidemic: its effect on total joint arthroplasty. J Arthroplasty 2007;22(6 Suppl 2):71–6.
19. Lotan Y, Bagrodia A, Roehrborn CG, et al. Are urologists fairly reimbursed for complex procedures: failure of 22 modifier? Urology 2008;72(3):494–7.
20. Huber TS, Carlton LM, O'Hern DG, et al. Financial impact of tertiary care in an academic medical center. Ann Surg 2000;231(6):860–8.
21. National health policy forum. edited; Office of Vice President for Research. Available at: http://www.nhpf.org. Accessed October 4, 2010.
22. The American Recovery and Reinvestment Act of 2009 Impact on DSH (Disproportionate Share Hospital). edited; U.S. Department of Health & Human Services. Available at: http://www.hhs.gov/recovery/. Accessed October 5, 2010.
23. National Health Policy Forum Publication, "The Basics-Medicaid Disproportionate Share Hospital (DSH) Payments." National Health Policy Forum. Available at: http://www.nhpf.org. Accessed October 22, 2010.

Index

Note: Page numbers of article titles are in **boldface** type.

A

Acetabular fractures, in obese patients
  causes of, 69
  open treatment of, **69–83**
    complications of, prevention of, 79–81
    general considerations in, 75
    intraoperative considerations in, 71
    literature related to, 77–79
    outcomes of, 77–79
    patient positioning for, authors' preferred
      practice, 71–75
    perioperative considerations in, 70–71
    surgical exposures in, authors' preferred
      practice, 75–77
  percutaneous treatment of, **55–67**
    case example, 60–62
    complications of, 60
    discussion, 62–66
    methods in, 55–56
    patient selection for, 55–56
    radiographic review in, 56–57
    results of, 60
    statistical analysis of, 58
    technique, 57–58
Anesthesia/anesthetics, for obese patients, 15
Ankle fractures. See also Ankle injuries.
  in obese patients, **45–53**
    prevalence of, 45
  prevalence of, 45
Ankle injuries, in obese patients, **45–53**
  epidemiology of, 45–46
  management of
    case example, 50–51
    immobilization in, 48–49
    outcomes, 50
    postoperative considerations in, 49–50
    surgical considerations in, 47–48
  perioperative considerations, 46–47
Arthritis, open treatment of acetabular/pelvic
  fractures in obese patients and, 81
Arthroplasty, in morbidly obese patients
  for knee arthrosis, 111–112
  total knee arthroplasty, 109–111
Arthrosis(es), knee, in morbidly obese patients,
  107–113. See also Knee arthrosis, in morbidly
  obese patients.

B

Bias, weight, in health care setting, 2
Blount disease, of tibia vara, in obese children,
  97–101
BMI. See Body mass index (BMI).
Body mass index (BMI), categories of, 2
Bracing, in spinal injury management in obese
  patients, 87

C

Children, obese, **95–105**
  increased incidence of, 95
  musculoskeletal trauma in, 95–102
    Blount disease of tibia vara, 97–101
    genu valgum, 101
    knee-related, 97
    SCFE, 101–102

D

Deep venous thrombosis (DVT), open treatment of
  acetabular/pelvic fractures in obese patients and,
  80–81
Diabetes, in morbidly obese patients, knee arthrosis
  with, treatment of, 111
DVT. See Deep venous thrombosis (DVT).

E

Elbow injuries, in obese patients, management of,
  13–14

F

Femoral neck fractures, ipsilateral, in obese patients,
  management of, 29
Femur shaft fractures, in obese patients
  diagnosis of, 22–23
  incidence of, 22
  management of, **21–35**
    fracture fixation in, 25–29
    interprosthetic fractures, 30–31
    ipsilateral femoral neck fractures, 29
    open fractures, 29–30

orthopedic.theclinics.com

Orthop Clin N Am 42 (2011) 129–132
doi:10.1016/S0030-5898(10)00100-8

Printed and bound by CPI Group (UK) Ltd, Croydon, CR0 4YY

03/10/2024

01040344-0018